SHATTERED

The Foul Body Odor that Almost Killed Me

by

Carry Wilson

DEDICATION

I want to thank GOD! This book is dedicated to anyone who suffers from any rare disorder, as they are challenging to diagnose and treat. I dedicate this book to anyone suffering from Trimethylaminuria/TMAU or any other body odor condition. This book is also dedicated to my family, the great city of New Orleans, Louisiana, and all the victims and survivors of hurricanes Katrina and Rita. Finally, I dedicate this book to Dr. George Preti who served as an analytical organic chemist at the Monell Chemical Senses Center for over forty years. Dr. Preti and a team of chemists led the fight for the cause, effects, origins, and treatment of TMAU. Rest in peace, Dr. George Preti (Dr. Preti/Dr. Pratt, 1944–2020).

TABLE OF CONTENTS

THE BEGINNING

1996, summer in Chicago. I was a twenty-year-old mother with a five-year-old daughter. We were at the beach with four of my best friends and their children. I stood in the sand, watching the children play and laugh. It was a beautiful, windy day. When a gust of wind blew by me, I smelled a musky scent coming off my body. I shouldn't have been musky because I bathed before we came to the beach.

Nevertheless, I put on more deodorant and joined my friends in the water. After about two hours of playing volleyball in the waist-deep water with my friends, one of them said, "It smells like fish out here." The other girls and I turned our noses up and looked around, but saw nothing.

Before we left the beach, I took another shower and put on some baby powder, deodorant, and clean clothes. We made it home at 8:00 p.m., and my daughter Sherry and I ate dinner, which my boyfriend had cooked. It was a humid night, so I opened the window and put Sherry to bed. Then I watched TV with my boyfriend, whom I had been in a relationship with for two years. As we sat on the bed watching TV, a cool breeze blew through the window, and again, I smelled the scent of musk coming off my body. I had taken a shower less than two hours before and had done nothing that would explain why I smelled overly musty. I thought to myself, *I need to switch my deodorant.*

The next day, Sherry and I met up with friends for a party at my best friend Daisy's house. My girls and I were hanging out outside on the porch when three guys we knew walked up and joined us.

We were all joking, laughing, and having fun when one guy shouted, "One of you bitches needs to take a douche! It smells like fish out here." Everybody looked at me. I started looking around on the ground as if I would see a dead fish or the source of the smell. Of course, the comment was disrespectful for him to make, but I grew up on the south side of Chicago in Englewood. Some guys say stupid things to be funny, so it wasn't a big deal. But I was embarrassed because I had been having some hygiene issues recently. I waited five minutes and then I left.

When I got home, it was 5:00 p.m. I cooked dinner and awaited my boyfriend's return from work. As expected, he came in, ate dinner, and took his bath for the night. Afterward, I calmly asked him to smell me. I put my chest up to his nose while I pulled my nightgown back. "What? You smell musty," he said.

I started to cry.

"Why are you crying?" he asked.

I told him I had just bathed and put on some deodorant and baby powder. "I should not be musty, but I am."

"Why don't you just take another bath?" he suggested. I thought about what that jerk had said earlier about someone needing to take a douche.

The next day, I went to see my doctor, whose name was Dr. Bloom. I thought the odor was coming from my vagina because it had an overly funky scent. I wondered if I possibly had an STD or a bacterial infection since I was having unprotected sex with my boyfriend.

I informed my doctor of my predicament, and he performed a vaginal exam and diagnosed me with a bacterial infection. He prescribed me fourteen pills to take over the next seven days.

I took them exactly as prescribed, but I continued to smell the odor. In fact, it seemed to be getting worse.

Ten days later, I returned to Dr. Bloom's office and told him I still had the odor. He gave me another prescription for the same medication.

In the meantime, I bathed daily and put on extra deodorant and baby powder. I also still spent time with my friends. Over the next six months, I would repeatedly hear comments from people saying that something smelled like shit or garbage whenever I was present. Sometimes, as soon as I walked up to some of my so-called friends, they would say, "Something stinks."

My boyfriend and I started growing apart. He did not understand what I was going through. He would always say, "It's not a big deal. You just need to switch your soap and deodorant," but I smelled terrible, and more people started to notice.

I visited Dr. Bloom four more times, complaining about my vaginal odor. I told him that more people were commenting about how I smelled. At my request, he tested me for HIV and ran other tests, all of which came back negative. On one of my visits with Dr. Bloom, he sat in a chair in the examination room, writing something in my folder. "If the odor continues...," he said as he took his finger and made a hand gesture, tapping his head as if to say the odor was in my head.

I did not overreact. "The odor is not in my head," I told him. "Other people smell me, too. Do you smell me?" I asked.

"I have never smelled an odor from you," he responded.

I did not know how to react to him saying he didn't smell an odor like feces coming from my body, one that I smelled every day. I also informed him on that visit that I had been feeling depressed. He said I should make an appointment with the nurse to see a psychiatrist.

"Okay," I said. Growing up in the ghetto, I thought only white people saw psychiatrists, and I didn't want to see one.

I continued seeing Dr. Bloom and two other doctors, who both said they did not smell an odor from me. Again, I did not react to these doctors saying they did not smell me, but I was overly concerned. How could they help me if they could not smell me, and why *couldn't* they smell me?

Two more months passed, and there was still an odor coming from my vagina. It was 7:00 p.m. and I was sitting on the back porch of my apartment building. I felt sad and I couldn't stop crying or thinking about people saying, "What's that smell?" or "Something stinks." I felt alone and scared. This was the first time I had felt that way.

My boyfriend had left four months earlier, but it was for the best. I hadn't wanted to have sex or be near a man while I smelled bad. For the first time in my life, I thought that if I weren't alive, I wouldn't feel the pain of having this odor; I wouldn't have to hear people commenting anymore. I began to have thoughts of killing myself to end all the embarrassment.

The next day, I called Dr. Bloom at 9:00 a.m. I told him I was feeling suicidal, and he told me to go to the hospital emergency room and talk to the nurse. I did exactly that.

I told the emergency room nurse I was feeling suicidal because I had an odor coming from my vagina. I was admitted and when I saw the doctor, he said he would run several tests to determine what was causing the odor. He returned six hours later and said he had good news: I only had a yeast infection.

I asked him, "Is that why I smell?" He said that women rarely have an odor when they have yeast infections. He prescribed me a one-dose treatment pill for yeast infections called Diflucan and said it should stop the odor. I left the hospital at 2:00 a.m.

I went home and went to bed, thinking the odor would be gone when I woke up because I'd taken the Diflucan. But at 9:30 a.m. I was home alone and still smelled an odor of trash coming from my vagina. I was in a daze; I wanted to kill myself.

Suddenly, I heard, "Carry, Carry!" I opened the window to see my father and Sherry standing outside. He told me he had errands to run for the day, so I needed to watch Sherry for several hours. My father had taken over parenting my daughter for the last seven months. I hadn't cooked for her or combed her hair since I'd developed the odor. All I cared about was stopping the odor. I had not told my daughter I loved her for several months. Being a mother to my daughter was too much for me to manage; I had to stop the odor first.

"Mama, I'm hungry," Sherry said when she entered the apartment.

"Make yourself something to eat," I said. Before my father took over as my daughter's parental guardian, he noticed that I let her cook hot dogs and eggs for herself. Sherry ironed her clothes for school and combed her hair, too. All I did was cry about the odor.

Sherry put two hot dogs on the stove. I was crying and had no strength to take care of her.

I was suicidal.

I walked back and forth through the apartment. I picked up a knife and imagined cutting my wrists and ending all the pain. My daughter noticed and started crying. "Mama, what is wrong? Why are you crying?" She asked. I told her to sit down, but she kept asking, "Mama, what's wrong?" I smacked her in the face so hard that her face turned red. I hugged her and apologized, but she continued asking why I was crying. She put so much pressure on me, and I could not handle her then. I felt scared. The knife was still in my hand. Before I hurt myself or Sherry, I needed to call the police.

I put the knife down and told Sherry to sit down and watch TV while I went to use the pay phone on the corner. I called the police. "My name is Carry Wilson," I told the police operator. "I am suicidal, and I have my daughter with me."

"Do not hang up the phone," she replied. "I am sending the police to you right now. Is your daughter next to you right now?"

"No, she's alone in the apartment," I said.

"It's going to be okay. The police are on their way," she assured me. "What color shirt do you have on?" she asked.

"Red," I replied. Standing at the pay phone, I prayed to God to help me. "You should be able to see the police car," the operator told me.

"I do," I said.

A police officer got out of the car. "Ms. Wilson?" he said. "Yes."

"Let's go get your daughter," he said.

We went upstairs and got Sherry. The officer took me and Sherry to Jackson Park hospital which was one mile from my apartment. Riding in the back of the police car, I felt numb to my surroundings. I could not feel my daughter's hug or hear her voice.

The officer took us straight to the emergency room at the back of the hospital, and I told the nurse I was suicidal. The nurse asked me if anybody could come to get my daughter, and I gave her the telephone number of Sherry's godparents. She then led me to a room with no windows or a bed.

She returned to the room three hours later and told me my daughter's godparents had picked her up and asked how I was doing. I saw a psychiatrist after another five hours.

"Ms. Wilson, my name is Dr. Sanders," he said. "How can I help you?"

"I have an odor coming from my vagina, and doctors keep saying there is no odor," I told him. "I cannot take it anymore.

People smell me and make mean comments whenever I'm present. Mean comments like, 'What's that smell?' or 'It stinks like a dead rat in here,'"

Dr. Sander asked me if I heard voices when no one was around, and I asked him if *he* heard voices when no one was around.

"Of course not! I am not crazy," I said.

"I didn't say you were crazy," he said. "I do not smell an odor from you right now." I cried and begged him to help me.

"How do you feel?" he asked.

"I just want to stop the odor," I said. "But I keep thinking about killing myself." Dr. Sander told me to get some rest and that he would give me some help.

I awoke to a knock on the door; it was the nurse. She brought me a sandwich and informed me they were waiting for an ambulance to transfer me to the University of Illinois Hospital. I asked her if she knew the time.

"Midnight," she replied. She told me my daughter's godparents had called to check on me again. "They wanted to know if we were releasing you from the hospital tonight. I told them I would tell you to call them when you could."

I did not want to call them; I felt embarrassed because I was suicidal and could not control my emotions. I felt like I was losing my mind. Doctors kept saying, "There is no odor coming from your vagina," but I had an odor. I knew they were wrong.

A knock on the door made me jump as I sat on the bed eating the sandwich. The nurse said, "The ambulance is here for you." I was shaking because it was cold in the hospital. My head hurt from crying all day, and I was still having thoughts of killing myself. The ride in the ambulance was scary. I had never been in an ambulance, so I hoped to return to the other hospital fast.

When we got to the hospital, the ambulance driver put me in a wheelchair, took me straight to the back of the emergency room, and handed a nurse my folder. They put me in another room with no windows or a bed. As she wrote in my folder, the nurse asked how I felt.

"I am feeling suicidal," I told her. "Why?" she asked.

"I have an odor coming from my vagina," I said. She looked up and directly into my eyes. I was embarrassed but felt so sad; I just wanted help.

She asked me how I would kill myself. I said I would cut my wrist or take pills as I started to cry. I did not like having thoughts like that.

"Why do you think you have this odor?" she asked.

"I don't know what is causing it," I said. I told her that people make mean comments about me because I have this odor, and doctors said they don't smell me. The nurse told me to change into a hospital gown and that the doctor would be in soon. She returned to the room two hours later, putting my clothes in a bag. I asked her if she smelled an odor when she entered the room.

"No," she said, "but your clothes have an odor."

Another five hours went by before the doctor entered the room. He was looking at a folder in his hand and said, "Hi, Ms. Wilson. I see here that you're suicidal because you think you have an odor coming from your vagina."

"I do not *think* I have an odor; I do," I said.

He asked me the same question the other doctor had asked: "Do you hear voices when no one else is around?"

I said no, but he asked me more questions. "Can you see things other people cannot?" "No."

"Who is the president?" "Bill Clinton."

"What day is it?" "Tuesday."

"What is your name?" "Carry Wilson."

"Where are you at right now?" "University of Illinois Hospital." "Why are you at the hospital?"

"I have a foul odor coming from my vagina, and doctors are saying there is no odor, and I just don't want to live anymore."

He asked me if I wanted to hurt myself. "Yes, to stop the pain, I replied."

He asked me if I was hungry. I said, "No."

He informed me that someone would come to pick me up soon. A few minutes later, a nurse took me straight to my room in the mental ward upstairs. I sat on the bed and looked around. The room had a chair, a bed, and a table with soap, toothpaste, a toothbrush, and hospital scrubs sitting on it. I also had a bathroom in my room. The room looked gloomy, but I felt safe. I no longer had to see my neighbors or hear their comments. I did not want to be in society anymore.

There was a knock on the door, and a nurse came in. "Hi," she said. "My name is Carol, and I'll be your nurse. You can come to the dayroom and eat breakfast."

I didn't know what to expect as I walked toward the dayroom. There was a long table with about twenty chairs up against it. There were two bookshelves full of books, two long couches, and a TV with a sign that read, "Do Not Turn TV To Jerry Springer."

As I stood there, patients walked past me and went to sit at the table. The nurse began calling their names so they could get their breakfast trays.

"Come sit over here," another woman patient said to me. I stood there in shock, thinking, *I do not need to be here. I am not crazy.* At that point, the other patients weren't acting crazy either. One patient walked past me and I saw at least twenty long scars across her arms, as if someone had cut her repeatedly. I was extremely uncomfortable but hungry, and the woman who told me to sit by her looked normal. I sat next to her and started eating. The girl with the scars on her arms asked me, "What is wrong with you? You look normal."

I told her I was feeling suicidal. She held her arms straight out across the table toward me and said her mother was a bitch and that she cut her arms up to hurt her mother.

"What did you cut your arms with?" I asked. She laughed and said, "A razor blade."

The woman who asked me to sit by her kicked my foot under the table while I talked to the girl who had cut herself. The girl got up to put her tray back on the food rack. "I was kicking you, trying to tell you not to talk to that girl," the woman said.

"Why?" I asked.

"That girl is crazy. She cut herself up to hurt her mother, but her mother is at home, and she is here with her arms all cut the fuck up. Who do you think is hurting, her or her mother?

What's your name?" she asked me. "Carry," I replied.

"I'm Teresa, she said. "You look too young to have any problems that would make you suicidal."

I told her, "I just don't feel well."

Teresa said her family put her in the hospital mental ward so they could get her SSI check every month. She was forty years old, but she looked at least sixty. She talked and acted normally, but I later realized she had a drug addiction.

When I returned my breakfast tray, a doctor approached me. "Carry Wilson?" he asked. "Yes, I replied."

"I need to speak to you in your room," he said. "My name is Dr. Rolston, and I will be your doctor." I asked him if he was a psychiatrist.

"Yes, I am," he replied. He asked me the same questions the other psychiatrist had asked.

But he also asked me to tell him about my childhood.

"No, I am not talking to you about my childhood because my childhood has nothing to do with why I am here," I said. "My childhood did not make me depressed. I am depressed because I have an odor coming from my vagina, and doctors keep saying there is no odor, and I do not want to live anymore," I cried.

"I want to give you some medicine to help you relax," said the doctor. "I am not taking any psychological medicine," I told him.

"Do you want me to help you?" he asked.

"Yes, I want you to find out why I have this odor coming from my vagina."

Dr. Rolston said, "Ms. Wilson, can I try to smell you?" I nodded. He circled me, sniffing my armpits and body. He said, "I cannot smell an odor from you." He told me I needed to get dressed for the group.

After showering and putting on my clothes, I sat on the bed. I started crying because yet another doctor had told me he could not smell me. I had seen many doctors, and they all said the same thing. They could not smell me. I sat on that bed thinking, *why don't the doctors take a piece of my tissue from my body and see if it is rotten or check if there is a dead baby in me?*

Something was wrong. I'd had this odor for several months and had seen doctor after doctor. They had checked for STDs and prescribed me antibiotics, but the odor never stopped. I could not understand why I needed antibiotics. I was not having sex; I smelled too bad. My so-called friends were some of the very people who commented about my odor, making me depressed. When I was on the bus or in a grocery store, people moved away from me and turned up their noses when they looked at me and coughed a lot around me. These incidents stopped being coincidences a long time ago. I always knew when people were reacting to my body odor. I sat on the bed crying until I heard a knock on the door and Carol, the nurse appeared.

"Come on, Carry. It's time for the group," she said. Walking toward her, I asked, "What is the group?"

"All the patients sit in a circle in the middle of the

dayroom," she explained. "We all get to know each other."

In the dayroom, I sat next to Teresa, who had saved me a seat next to her.

"Hi, everybody," Carol began. She pointed to a man and said, "This is Kent, and he is a nurse on this floor as well."

"Everybody who came in this morning or last night, when I point to you, stand up and tell us your name and why you are here," Kent said. He then pointed to a guy who stood up.

"Hi, my name is Greg, and I'm depressed," he said by way of introduction. "Hi Greg," everyone responded in unison.

Kent pointed to a girl. She stood up and spoke loudly. "Hi. My name is Erica, and I do not want to be here, but it is okay. God will take care of me and all of us."

"Okay, Erica, you can sit down now," Carol said, but Erica kept talking. Kent got up, grabbed Erica by the hand, and led her out of the dayroom. Carol told me to wait until Kent came back before I spoke.

Kent came back after ten minutes without Erica and pointed to me. I stood up and said, "Hi. My name is Carry, and I am depressed and suicidal."

Everyone said, "Hi, Carry!"

The group was a promising idea. It gave patients a chance to talk about their feelings. We all wanted to improve so we could return to society, be better people, and lead everyday lives.

After the group, I called my daughter and my father. It felt good to hear Sherry's voice.

My father asked if I wanted him to visit me. I told him no; I did not want him to see me in a mental hospital.

Afterward, I ate lunch and talked to a counselor for twenty minutes about how I felt. I told her I felt safe in the mental ward. After the counselor left, I read medical books I found on the shelves until 5:00 p.m., when it was time for dinner. After dinner, I watched TV.

It was 7:00 p.m. when Kent walked into the dayroom with a tray of food and set it on the table. Erica came in, walking slowly behind Kent. Her eyes looked closed, but they were open. She waved and said, "Heeeeeeeeyyyyyy, everybody," with a slur like she was in slow motion. I watched her closely as she sat there eating her food. She drooled uncontrollably and fell asleep while eating. I became concerned about Erica. After seeing her so vocal that morning, she was acting like she was a zombie.

As we all looked at Erica, Teresa whispered in my ear, "If you keep telling these doctors you want to kill yourself, they're going to put you on some fucked up medicine like that." She pointed to Erica. Seeing Erica behave like that confirmed my belief that psychological drugs turn sane people crazy. I knew I would never take any psychological medication. Erica remained in that zombielike state until the day I left the mental ward.

The next morning, Dr. Rolston saw me in my room. He asked if I still smelled the odor. I said yes.

"I want you to get a CT scan today after lunch," he said.

After I got the CT scan, he came into the dayroom and told me that he needed to speak to me in my room.

When we got there, he told me, "Your CT scan showed no abnormalities, and I want to start you on medication to help you stop thinking about the odor."

"What is this medicine for?" I asked Dr. Rolston.

"It will treat the delusions you have that make you think you have body odor," he explained. "You have a chemical imbalance."

I asked him, "What if I have an odor and you're wrong? If I take this medicine, isn't it going to cause a chemical imbalance that was not there before?" I honestly thought that if I took medication for delusions, which I did not have, the medication would somehow chemically change my brain and lead to an imbalancc. Also, I knew I had the odor, and the doctor was wrong.

Dr. Rolston avoided answering my question. Instead he said, "That will not happen; this medicine will help you."

"I would feel much better if you could just send me to a specialist, not a gynecologist," I said. "Since my body odor started, all I have seen are gynecologists, and they could not stop the odor." In 1996, I thought all doctors were the same, but after reading books in the hospital, I realized there are diverse medical fields and specialties. I begged him to let me see if one more doctor could help me. He said he would look into getting me the name and address of a doctor before they discharged me.

For the next two days, I felt better. I felt ready to go home to see my daughter and a new type of doctor. I had been in the ward for six days and five nights.

On my last day in the ward, Dr. Rolston came to see me before breakfast and asked me how I felt.

"I'm eager to see the new doctor you will refer me to." I said. He asked me if I still smelled the odor.

"Yes," I said.

"Would you just consider taking the medicine?" he asked.

"No," I told him. "I am going to be okay." I was hopeful the new doctor would help me eliminate the odor.

I ate breakfast and talked to Teresa. She told me she had been in the ward for twenty days because she would not let the doctors tell her what to do.

"Good luck if I never see you again," I told her.

Carol finally arrived at noon and said, "Carry, it's time to go."

I hugged Teresa and went to the front desk of the ward. The discharge nurse handed me a referral to Dr. Sarah Landry's clinic and a bag with a toothbrush, toothpaste, water jug, wash pan, and a token to catch the bus. As I got on the elevator, Carol ran up to me and tried to hand me the prescription for that medicine.

"No, I'm not taking that," I said.

"Carry, please, just in case you need it," she persisted. I shook my head as the elevator door closed. When I got outside, I felt the wind against my skin and smelled the air. It felt so good.

As soon as I got home and opened the door to my apartment, a horrible scent assaulted me. My apartment smelled like mildew. I almost cried but was hopeful the new doctor would stop the odor. I called my father and told him that I was home. I asked him to let me speak to Sherry.

"Mama are you at home?" she said over the phone.

"Yes. Granddaddy is going to bring you home soon," I said. Talking to my daughter always made me feel better about living.

I called the doctor's office from the pay phone on the corner and got an appointment for the next day at 10:00 a.m. I went back to my apartment and opened all the windows. I mopped the floors with half a gallon of bleach; I would rather the apartment smelled like too much bleach than my odor, which smelled like urine, trash, or rotten food. People said different things about how I smelled.

Then I fried some chicken and made rice. It had been several months since I had cooked dinner for my daughter. It felt good to act normally for a change.

When my father and daughter arrived, my father

immediately came in, made Sherry a plate of food, and told her to sit down and eat it.

"Your mother and I are stepping out into the hallway to talk," he told her. I did not know what my father would say. We stepped into the hallway and left the door ajar. My father spoke very seriously and told me that I needed to get through whatever I was going through, get a job, and care for Sherry. He said he was getting older and could not care for Sherry daily; if she were a boy, it would be easier for him to run around with her. He added, "Some people just smell how they smell." That destroyed me. He told me, "Those doctors spent years in medical school. They have licenses and degrees, and you are trying to tell them they're wrong." I respect my father very much. He knows I love life, love to work, and want to succeed. My father is the person who taught me to stand up for what I believe in. So it hurt when he told me to get over the fact that I smelled like shit and to go back to work no matter what.

All I could say was, "Daddy, the doctors are wrong. Something has gone wrong in my body." I told him I was going to the doctor the next day and would be okay. My father shook his head in disappointment that I was continuing to see doctors, but this was my life. I asked him if he could loan me money until I got my welfare check; I needed bus fare to get to the doctor. I also asked him if he could watch Sherry for me the following day until I got back from the doctor.

He said with frustration, "I am going to give you this money, but this time, if this doctor says there is nothing wrong, you need to get a job and start being a mother to Sherry. School starts soon. She needs school supplies and clothes." I took twenty dollars out of his hand.

"Thank you, and the doctor will help me this time," I said.

After a few hours, Sherry and my father left and I went to

bed extra early. I awoke at 8:00

a.m. I took my bath and headed down the hallway to the exit. There were fifteen other apartments in the building. Walking down the hall, two other women who lived in the building passed me. "Good morning," I said.

They said hello, and then one said, "This whole hallway smells like mildew."

As I turned to go down the stairs, I stopped and almost cried. I put towels at the bottom of my apartment's front and back doors to stop my odor from entering the hallway.

I made it to the doctor's office at 9:20 a.m. I filled out the patient history forms and waited forty minutes before the nurse called my name and led me into the exam room. The doctor came in a few minutes later.

"Hi, Ms. Wilson," she said. "I am Dr. Landry." She looked like a good doctor. She looked at my folder and said, "I see you have an odor coming from your vagina."

"Yes," I said.

"Do you have any itching or discharge?" she asked. "No," I said.

"What type of douche do you use?" she asked. I started crying. She put her hand on my knee and asked, "Why are you crying?"

"You are just like the other doctors," I said. "Every day, I wash my body with soap and water. I douche once a month. The doctors have been giving me antibiotics for several months, and the odor will not stop."

"Ms. Wilson," she said, "I see here you said the other doctors said they did not smell you. I do not smell an odor from you, but that does not mean you do not have an odor." She asked me what types of food I ate, informing me that certain foods could sometimes contribute to body odor. "The odor comes out through your sweat."

"Just regular food," I said.

"I will tell you what I will do," she said. "I will do a vaginal exam and run some tests after the exam. I want you to douche with the cleanser Betadine and use Arm & Hammer deodorant. Get some Arm & Hammer baking soda, and if you do not wear pantyliners now, start wearing them. Put a little Arm & Hammer baking soda in your vaginal area." She told me not to worry so much. "Everything is going to be okay. I will see you in two weeks."

When I left Dr. Landry's office, I was hopeful that all these hygiene steps would stop my odor. I stopped at the store and bought everything she had told me to purchase. That night, after I bathed, I douched with the cleanser, put on the deodorant, and sprinkled some Arm & Hammer baking soda on the panty-liner before I put it on. I noticed the odor was not foul anymore; it was fresh. I wanted the odor to stop, so I made myself believe that the odor was gone. I kept smelling myself all day, and I did not smell foul. I did not stop eating the food I had always eaten.

It was not like Dr. Landry said. "Carry. If you eat spicy food, your body will have an odor."

I got my welfare check and had to buy food and my daughter's school clothes and supplies. I bought some more hygiene products, and I felt better. My father paid my rent and light bill, and I felt confident enough to look for a job. It took less than two weeks to find a job at a hotel as a housekeeper.

I saw Dr. Landry one more time before I started working. I told her the odor was not foul anymore. She hugged me and said she was happy I felt much better. I informed her I would like to get a procedure that would stop me from having a menstrual cycle. I told her I was worried I would have to use extra hygiene products every month when my cycle came, so I wanted to stop my menstrual cycle altogether.

"You are too young," she said. "You should not do anything

drastic to stop your monthly cycle. Let me give you a pregnancy test right now, and if it is negative, I will start you on birth control pills. When you are supposed to stop the old pack and start on the new pack of pills, keep taking them, and your period will stop." I asked her if that was safe to do. "Yes, it will stop your period," she replied.

I started work four days later. On my first day of work, everything was okay. On the second day of work, as I walked down the hotel hallway and passed another housekeeper, she bent the top half of her body away from me as she passed. I'd had no problem the day before so I did not overreact to her odd behavior. However, when all the housekeepers went downstairs to the lunchroom for lunch, I sat alone at a table that could have fit at least five other people; they all chose to stand.

While eating my lunch, I heard a male housekeeper tell another housekeeper, "You need to tell Tanya (the housekeeping supervisor) that the twelfth-floor stinks. It smells like shit up there." I immediately panicked; I had worked on the twelfth floor on my first day. I stood up and went straight to the pay phone in the hotel lobby.

I called Dr. Landry's office and told the nurse I needed to speak to the doctor. I started crying uncontrollably.

"Ms. Wilson, what's wrong?" Dr. Landry asked.

"This odor is still here," I said. "Nothing has changed. People are still talking about me.

Please help me." I felt like I would drop to the floor; my knees felt weak.

"I don't know what to tell you," Dr. Landry said. "Your test results were negative. There is no reason you should have body odor. As a gynecologist, I have done everything I can for you. The only thing I can think of doing is talking to a dermatologist to see if they have ever heard of anything like this." I could not stop crying. I had never seen a dermatologist. She asked me if I was feeling depressed or suicidal.

"No," I replied. "I just want to stop this odor."

Dr. Landry told me she would talk to the dermatologist the following day and that I should call her at 11:00 a.m. the next day.

"Thank you," I said, wiping my tears before returning to work. I was extremely uncomfortable. Whenever my supervisor came close to me to check my room chart, I became physically nervous. I could not wait to get off work. When I clocked out, I said goodnight to everybody. Neither my supervisor nor coworkers said, "Goodbye" or "We will see you tomorrow." I knew they heard me speak to them. I never understood why people disliked me; I smelled bad, but I was still a good person. I left work in tears.

When I got home, my father and daughter were there. My father looked at me and said, "You've been crying. You aren't going back to work, are you?"

"I don't know," I said.

That night, when I lay down to sleep, I looked at my daughter. I thought I could not care for you while I was like this. I could feel myself getting depressed and having suicidal again. I lay in bed and decided I was not returning to the hotel. I would rather talk to the dermatologist with Dr. Landry and tell them directly about my vaginal odor. I did not know what a dermatologist was, but I knew they were not gynecologists.

The next morning, my father woke me up at 6:00 a.m. He asked me if I was going to work. "Yes, I am." I lied to him so he would watch Sherry. I did not want to have to be a mother to her that day. I know that sounds bad, but I was an emotional wreck.

When my father and Sherry left, my father yelled at me, "Stop putting towels under the door! No one has a problem with the way you smell. No one says anything to me about you smelling bad." My father thought people would walk up to him and say, "Your daughter Carry smells terrible," and since that didn't happen, he assumed there was no problem.

I left home at 9:30 a.m. When the bus made it to the hospital district, I got off at a stop I wouldn't normally get off at because I wanted to kill some time. It was only 10:00 a.m. Dr.

Landry had told me to call her back at 11:00 a.m., but I wanted to give her time to talk to the dermatologist.

As I walked down the street looking at the buildings, I saw a sign in front of a gigantic building on Polk Street that read, "The University of Chicago Health and Science Library." The words "Health and Science" made me want to enter the library. I had always thought doctors needed to examine a piece of my tissue under a microscope to figure out what was causing the odor.

I approached the receptionist. I was so embarrassed, but I asked her if the library had any books on female body odors. She clicked a few buttons on the computer and said, "No, not under that title." She offered, "Let me try a different title." She clicked more and said, "We have a book titled *The Human Body Odor*." She wrote down the row and floor. I could not find the book, but the librarian helped me.

On the front of the book, in big letters, was the title, *The Human Body Odor*, and on the back of the book was a small paragraph: "The etiology and treatment of sweat gland surgery, hair loss, and body odor." I immediately became intrigued. Was the cure for my vaginal odor in this book? I turned to the index. There were contents for body odor and the smell of feces, body odor and bacterial infections, case reports of people with a condition called bromhidrosis (of course, I could not pronounce the conditions correctly), and testing methods for body odor.

I turned to the section on body odor and the smell of feces; it documented how patients with bromhidrosis would complain of smelling like feces. I turned to the case reports, and one case stood out. A nineteen-year-old female complained of having a foul body odor. She complained about how people commented on her body odor, turned their noses up, or opened windows when she was present. The dermatologists who treated her were the authors of the book. They stated that there was no objective odor present; however, these dermatologists understood the condition and knew there were testing methods other than smelling the odor from the patient. The dermatologists performed sweat gland removal surgery on this patient.

I almost fell to the floor, crying. As I continued to read, I became convinced I had this condition. I concluded that the odor was also coming from my armpits and between my breasts. The odor was not inside my vagina but coming from the vaginal wall. I knew I needed to get my sweat glands removed.

I looked up at the clock; it was 11:45 a.m. I was late. I had to get this book to Dr. Landry and the dermatologist. I could show them that a person could have a body odor that some people smell and others do not. I had learned from the book that everyone's perception of smell is different; what smells foul to me may not smell foul to someone else. I smelled horrible. How could any doctor smell me and not perceive the odor as foul? I never really understood completely. But as doctors, Dr. Landry and the dermatologist would understand these concepts.

As I left the library, I stopped at the check-out desk. I handed the book to the clerk and told her I wanted to check the book out. I pulled out my state ID and gave it to the librarian.

When she looked at my ID, she told me that I had to be a student or a doctor at the hospital or university to check the book out.

I told her, "I will just ask my doctor to return and get the book." The clerk made me a copy of the front and back of the book. I thought it would be a good idea to show Dr. Landry a copy of the book's title and the paragraph on the back. I was in overdrive to show her I had discovered what was wrong with me!

I made it to the clinic and told Dr. Landry's nurse I needed to speak with Dr. Landry. "We are busy today. Do you have an appointment?" she asked.

"Please tell Dr. Landry I must see her immediately," I pleaded. I waited twenty minutes, but it seemed like an hour.

"Ms. Wilson, I can see you now," Dr. Landry said. When we got into the examination room, I gave her the copies of the front and back of the book. As she read, I anxiously told her about bromhidrosis! I told her about the book, especially about sweat gland removal surgery.

"This is some useful information," she said. "I am so proud of you." I told her, "I cannot check the book out, but you can."

She told me I needed to see my primary care physician and tell him about the book.

"What about the dermatologist you spoke with today?" I asked her. "The authors of the book are dermatologists."

She said, "I have not spoken with the dermatologist today, but you can go upstairs and make an appointment in the dermatology department."

I left her office with no medical records to show the dermatologist. I went upstairs to the dermatology department. The nurse asked if I had a referral after I signed in.

"No," I said, "but my doctor told me I could just come up here and make an appointment."

The nurse said, "You need a referral from your primary care doctor to see a dermatologist."

I said "Ok," and thanked her. I did not like my primary care doctor. Dr. Bloom had made it clear that he did not smell an odor coming from me and thought I needed to see a psychiatrist. But I had no choice but to get a referral from him. I had to see him again.

The next morning, my father and daughter came home early. I told my father I had a doctor's appointment. My father said, with anger in his voice, "You need to get this girl ready for school." I hadn't noticed that school was starting soon.

"Daddy, I just need you to help me a little longer until I can find out what is wrong with me," I said. I knew I could not show him the papers on bromhidrosis or tell him about the book. He would say I was chasing a ghost again.

My father told me he had spoken with my sister Candice in New Orleans and asked her to consider letting my daughter Sherry live with her for a little while.

I asked him, "Did she say yes?"

"Would you let her go?" my father asked.

"Hell yeah," I said. My daughter put too much pressure on me, and I was an emotional wreck, but I had hope again. I had found a book that explained what was wrong with me. No doctor could tell me I did not have a body odor.

I kissed Sherry and told her I would see her later. I made it to my primary care doctor's office at 9:00 a.m. The nurse led me into the exam room, and Dr. Bloom came in a few minutes later.

"Hi, Ms. Wilson. How can I help you?"

"I need a referral to see a dermatologist. I need to get my sweat glands removed," I said. "A dermatologist will not remove your sweat glands," he told me.

"Whatever," I said, dismissively. "I need to get a referral from you." "Ms. Wilson, I do not see a reason to refer you to a dermatologist." I lost it. I cursed and cried.

Dr. Bloom's nurse came into the exam room and said, "Ms. Wilson, you need to lower your voice." But I continued to curse at Dr. Bloom.

She said, "I think you should leave, Ms. Wilson."

Walking toward the door, I said, "Dr. Bloom, are you going to give me the fucking referral or not?"

"There is no reason for seeing a dermatologist," he said.

I left Dr. Bloom's office in despair. I went to the first payphone I saw and called my HMO medical insurance provider.

"My primary care doctor refused to refer me to a dermatologist," I told the HMO phone agent. "I am depressed and suicidal because I have a foul odor coming from my body. The only specialists who can help me are the dermatologists who have written a book explaining my medical condition."

"Do you think you will hurt yourself?" the operator asked me. "I just need to see a dermatologist," I pleaded.

"I am scared to let you off the phone," she said. "I can feel the pain in your voice. If you have problems with your current doctor, you must switch your primary care doctor, which will take about two weeks. If you feel you will hurt yourself before then, please go to an emergency room."

"Okay," I said.

When I got home, some of my neighbors were sitting outside in front of the apartment building.

"Hi, Carry. Come and chill out with us," one of them said. I kept walking straight past them and did not even look at them.

When I made it up to my apartment, I felt depressed and could not stop crying. I felt like I was going to throw up. I had to talk to myself. I did not want to become depressed; the doctors would admit me back into the psychiatric ward. I told myself it was going to be all right. *Stay strong, Carry, you can make it.* I always asked God to stay with me. *You will get the help you need.*

When Sherry and my father came home that night, I had to stop crying and put on a phony smile, but I wanted to be alone. My father told me he was taking my daughter to New Orleans because school had started there, and he wanted Sherry to get caught up. He said they would leave in a week. He insisted I call my sister Candice to thank her for letting Sherry come and stay with her.

I went to my neighbor Lewis's apartment and asked him to let me call my sister. I paid Lewis to let jobs I had applied for leave me messages on his answering service, so he sometimes let me use his phone.

"Hey, little sister, I miss you so much," my sister hollered. We had not seen each other in about three years. We had been close when I was a little girl; my father would be at work, and my sister was my mother, sister, and best friend. "Carry, I am worried about you," she said.

I told her, "I have a medical condition, but I am getting help soon, and I will be down there to get Sherry back as soon as I get cured."

My sister asked me to move to New Orleans, but I told her I loved living in Chicago.

Chicago is a great city with many great opportunities. If a person takes advantage of those opportunities, they could become successful. Besides, my first love, Evan, lived in Chicago. But I had to admit that I was both happy and sad that my daughter was leaving. I was relieved Sherry would be in a safe environment and I could finally focus all my energy and time on removing my sweat glands.

When my father returned to Chicago after dropping my daughter off in New Orleans, he said Sherry was crying when he left, and he told her I would be there to see her soon. "Carry, whatever you are doing, get it done, and get your ass back to work," my father said.

I finally received my new doctor's name and address: Dr. White. I called the clinic and made an appointment for the next day. I was so excited about the new appointment that I watched TV for the first time in several months. I disliked watching TV; I disliked seeing people laughing and enjoying life. But I was so excited about seeing a new doctor that I felt well enough to watch

TV and laugh along with the sitcoms.

Someone outside yelled, "Carry, Carry!" while I was watching TV. I did not look out the window, but I recognized the voice of one of my so-called best friends, Daisy, whom I had known for over fifteen years. I turned the TV down and went to hide in my bathroom, just in case one of my neighbors let Daisy in through the front door of the building. I did not want to let her into my apartment; she would return to my old neighborhood and tell everyone we knew that I still smelled bad. On more than one occasion, Daisy had made comments around me that something smelled like garbage. I would not let her humiliate me. I did not consider her my friend anymore.

Finally, after twenty minutes, I came out of the bathroom. She was gone. I went to bed early again to make it to my 10:00 a.m. appointment with my new doctor.

I made it to the doctor's office at 9:30 a.m. I wrote on the patient information form that I needed a referral to see a dermatologist. The nurse called me and led me to an examination room. Dr. White came in ten minutes later, looking at the information in my folder.

"Hi, Ms. Wilson," he said, "I am Dr. White. Why do you need to see a dermatologist?" "I have a foul odor coming from my body," I said. "At least six doctors have said they

don't smell the odor from me. *The Human Body Odor* is a book I found. I relate to this condition, bromhidrosis, that is in the book." I handed him copies of the back and front of the book.

After reading the copies, Dr. White told me to lie on the table so he could examine me, which consisted of him pushing down on my stomach and asking me if I felt pain. He told me to sit up, and he looked down my throat and into my ears. "Ms. Wilson, I do not smell an odor from you," he said.

I said, "In this book, the dermatologist did not smell the odor from the patient, but they still removed her sweat glands. There are other testing methods besides smelling an odor."

"Where is this book?" he asked.

"The University Library on Polk Street." You are a doctor; you can get the book." I told him again, "I need to see a dermatologist."

I was wearing a miniskirt and had put baby oil on my legs. "Ms. Wilson, nothing is wrong with you." Dr. White said after examining me. "Look at your legs; you look good."

I started crying. "I don't care how good I look. I have a foul odor coming from my body." "Why are you crying?" he asked.

"I need to see a dermatologist!"

"I am not giving you a referral, but I will get the book and read it," he told me. I cried so much that Dr. White asked me if I was depressed.

"Yes!" I yelled. "Doctor after doctor keeps telling me I do not have a body odor, and I do."

He gave me a tissue and said he would perform a pelvic examination to see if I had a bacterial infection that could cause a minor odor.

"I do not need a pelvic exam," I said. "I do not have sex with anyone, and the odor is not minor. As a doctor, you should know that people with bacterial infections do not have body odor."

"Ms. Wilson, please stop trying to be a doctor, and since you are refusing to let me examine you for a bacterial infection, I will get the book and give you a return appointment for two weeks." He asked me the name of the book again.

"I just showed you the paper with the book's title," I said as I cried uncontrollably. "Ms. Wilson, please lie down until you calm down, and I will give you a return appointment for one week."

"No, I am leaving," I said.

As soon as I got home, I closed all the curtains in the apartment, went into the bathroom, and closed the door. I turned off the lights and got under the bathroom sink in a fetal position. I cried. I felt all alone and scared. I had intense thoughts about committing suicide. There were a lot of reasons to kill myself. I started to think Dr. Bloom was calling these other doctors and telling them that I was crazy and that they shouldn't help me. Why else would every doctor I see keep saying that I did not have a body odor? I wanted to die.

I awoke to a knock on my front door. I did not want to answer it, but I did. My legs were stiff as I got up from under the bathroom sink. It was my neighbor, Lewis, from downstairs. "A doctor is on the phone for you," he yelled.

I opened the door. "What time is it?" I asked. He said it was 4:00 p.m. "I will be right down," I told him.

For four hours, I had slept under the bathroom sink. When I picked up the phone, I didn't know which doctor was calling.

"Hello?" It was Dr. White, the doctor I had seen earlier that day.

"Hi, Ms. Wilson," he said. "I have not been able to stop thinking about you since you left the clinic this morning. I want to get you some help. You need to go to the emergency room at Touro Hospital and ask for me."

I did not know what type of help he thought he could give me, but I knew I needed help. When I got to the hospital emergency room, I asked the nurse for Dr. White.

"What is your name?" she asked. "Carry Wilson," I replied.

"You can come with me," she said.

We got on the elevator and got off on the fourth floor. She led me to a regular hospital room with a bed and a TV. "You can put on that hospital gown," she said, pointing toward the bed.

I asked her what was going on. She told me Dr. White would be in to see me soon. I sat on the bed and started crying. I still felt suicidal.

The nurse came back into the room an hour later. "Are you

okay?" she asked. I said no.

"Come with me," she said, leading me to the bathroom in the room. "Go put on your gown and lay down in the bed. I will get you some apple juice." I put on the gown and lay down on the bed. The nurse brought me some crackers and apple juice, but I did not eat them. I fell asleep.

I awoke to a knock on the door. It was Dr. White.

"Hi, Ms. Wilson. The nurse told me you were crying." He asked me questions as he wrote in a folder. He asked me if I still thought I had a body odor; I said yes. He asked me if I was still feeling depressed; I said yes.

"Are you having thoughts of hurting yourself?" he asked. I said yes. "I was worried about you when you left my office," he told me.

"Is that why you brought me here?" I asked him.

"Yes," he said. I hoped he had brought me back to help me with my body odor. "I just want the odor to stop," I said.

He asked, "When you think about hurting yourself, what do you think you will do?" "I don't know," I said. I did not want to talk to him.

"I want to give you something to help you sleep," he told me.

"No, I am not taking any medicine," I said. "The medicine will help you relax," he said.

I said no, and he left the room. Throughout the night, Dr. White returned to the room with papers for me to sign. I didn't read the papers I was signing.

Dr. White said, "We are waiting to transfer you by ambulance to the University of Illinois Hospital."

"To the mental ward?" I asked.

"You will get the help you need there," he replied.

I did not care; I wanted to go back to the mental ward. I

wanted to be away from the world again.

At 4:00 a.m., I arrived at the University of Illinois Hospital. They took me straight to the mental ward on the same floor but put me in a different room. I lay in bed, and a psychiatrist came into the room a few hours later.

"Ms. Wilson, I know you came into the hospital this morning and are sleepy, but I need to speak with you," he said. I got out of bed and sat on a chair.

"I will be your doctor," he said. "My name is Dr. Walsh." He handed me a banana and apple juice. He asked questions while writing in a folder. "Why are you feeling suicidal?"

"I have a foul odor coming from my body. Doctors keep saying there is no odor, but I smell the odor, and other people around me smell the odor; I cannot even keep a job because of the odor," I told him. "I am poor. I cannot even take care of myself," I continued.

He asked me, "What started the odor?"

"Like I told the other doctors, I don't know. But I found a book about a condition that causes a person to have a foul body odor, and I relate to the condition one hundred percent. The book has all the answers in it. You are a university doctor; you can get the book this morning. The library is less than two blocks from here."

He asked me the book's name and wrote it down. "Did something happen right before the odor started?" he asked.

"No," I said. "In the book, it's a medical condition." I asked if he could smell me. "No, I do not smell you," he said.

"I need to see a dermatologist because the book's authors are dermatologists, and they understand the condition," I explained.

"I want you to get a CT scan later," he said.

"I already had one done the first time I was here," I explained, "and whatever it showed, the doctor still said I didn't have a body odor. He was wrong, so I don't see the point in a CT scan."

"Well, I want to get another one done. You can go eat breakfast now, and then I want you to get some rest," he said, leaving my room.

As I walked out of my room, going to the dayroom to eat breakfast, I passed Carol. "Oh, hi, Carry," she said. "You're back. I hope you feel better soon."

While in the mental ward this time, I decided I would not talk to the other patients. I would read books and stay in my room as much as possible.

After eating breakfast, I lay down until Carol came into my room. "Carry, you need to get a CT scan now," she said.

Several hours later, after I had the CT scan, Dr. Walsh came into my room, writing in my folder and asking me several questions. "Where are you at right now?" he asked.

"In the hospital mental ward," I said.

"Are you a man or a woman?" "A woman."

"What time of day is it?" "Afternoon."

He held up two fingers. "How many fingers do you see?" "Two."

"What brought you to the ward?"

"I am depressed and suicidal because I have a condition that makes me have a foul body odor.

"Do you smell the odor right now?" "Yes."

I informed Dr. Walsh that I live on the third floor of my apartment building, and because of my body odor, I always open all the windows to let the fresh air in. Flies are attracted to my foul scent, so my apartment has a lot of flies in it.

He immediately looked up at me. "You see flies?" he asked. I was fucked. "No, there are real flies," I said.

He didn't answer but wrote something in my folder. The more I talked to doctors, the more they seemed convinced that I had a mental illness. I did not have a mental illness. Flies were attracted to my foul body odor in the same way they were attracted to the scent of rotten food or dog feces.

"I want to start you on some medicine to help you stop thinking you have a body odor," Dr. Walsh said.

"No," I said. "I do have a body odor, and I will never take any psychiatric medication."

"I cannot help you if you do not let me," he said. "You need to think about taking the medicine. If not for yourself, then for your daughter. I see here you have a daughter. The medicine will stop your delusions that are causing you to believe you have a body odor."

I asked if he had ever met another patient with a mental illness who specifically stated that they had a body odor. "Is this even a sickness?" I asked. "Why would I say I had body odor if I'm delusional? Wouldn't I say I see fifty people when there is just one person? I answered all your questions right, so I cannot be delusional."

"You have a chemical imbalance that makes you think you have an odor coming from your body. I want you to take the medicine, and we can help you get some financial help."

"What kind of financial help?" I asked.

"You can get a monthly check to help you care for yourself and your daughter," he said. "A check for what?" I asked.

"Your mental disability," he replied.

"I do not want to get a check every month; I want to work!" I growled. "You said you cannot care for yourself or your daughter," he said.

"Because of the odor!" I yelled at him. "If you help me see a dermatologist, I can eliminate this odor. I will not sit at home waiting for a check every month. I have goals." I told Dr. Walsh I did not want to live off the government, especially since I could work, and I wanted to work. I walked out of the room. I didn't want to talk to him anymore.

The next morning, as I ate breakfast, instead of Dr. Walsh, a counselor came to see me. "Ms. Wilson, if you do not take the medicine Dr. Walsh is trying to start you on, you will not get better," she said. "You are going around saying you see flies. None of the doctors can smell you. I am sitting beside you right now and do not smell you. Do you believe you are right and everyone else is wrong?" she asked.

"Yes, I am right, and they are wrong!" I told her.

She shook her head. "You must let the doctors help you."

The following day, after I ate breakfast, I called my father and told him I was in the mental ward again. He said he was worried I had not come home the day before, and none of my neighbors could recall the last time they had seen me. My father wasted no time telling me, again, that I was wasting my life. "I hope you have a way to pay your bills," he said. "Do you think I will pay your bills every month while you run around in hospitals acting crazy?" I did not want to, but I hung up on him. He was making me feel bad. I would tell him my minutes ran out on the phone, which was why the phone hung up.

I respect my father too much to disrespect him, but I needed him to help me fight against these doctors, and he was unwilling to do so. My father loved me, but he was from the old school. If the doctor said your face hurts because you are ugly, my father would believe whatever the doctor said. My father not having my back in this situation was scary for me. My father taught me to fight for what I believed in and use common sense in my everyday life, which was what I was doing. I smelled a foul odor coming from my body, and the doctors kept saying the odor was not there. My common sense told me they were wrong, so how could they help me?

Until I found a doctor who could smell me, I would keep fighting.

Later that morning, after group, I called Dr. Landry at her

clinic. I told her I was in the hospital's mental ward. I asked her to call Dr. Walsh and tell him I was not crazy. "Tell him you saw me before and about the book and the surgery," I pleaded with her.

"I will call him and tell him I have seen you as a patient," she said. Dr. Landry was my only hope.

Later that day, Dr. Walsh came in for the second of his three visits with me. I informed him that Dr. Landry would call him that day to tell him about the book and the sweat gland surgery and let him know I was not crazy.

"Okay, Ms. Wilson," he said. "Are you going to take the medicine today?" I said, "No!"

He asked me if I was feeling suicidal.

"I feel a little better now that I know Dr. Landry will call you," I said. "The medicine will stop you from having any feelings of suicide," he said. I walked away from him. I just wanted him to talk to Dr. Landry.

Later that afternoon, I called Dr. Landry. It was Friday, and Dr. Landry needed to call before the end of the day. I knew I would see Dr. Walsh for the last time between 4:00 and 5:00

p.m. I pleaded with her to call him before the day was over, and she said she had not called him yet but would do so at 4:30 p.m.

Dr. Walsh finally came to see me at 4:30 p.m. Before he could say anything, I asked him, "Did Dr. Landry call you yet?"

He said, "No, she has not called," and I immediately went and called her on the patient's phone.

"Dr. Landry, here is Dr. Walsh," I said. "Please talk to him." I handed the phone receiver to Dr. Walsh. I could not wait for him to get off the phone.

He talked to Dr. Landry for about ten minutes. Dr. Walsh hung up the phone and wrote something in my folder.

He said, "Let's go to your room and talk."

When we got to my room, he told me Dr. Landry told him I was harassing her. "She said she saw you in her clinic but did not smell an odor coming from you. Ms. Wilson, if you call Dr. Landry again, I will have no choice but to put you on phone restriction." My mouth dropped open. I could not believe that Dr. Landry had abandoned me. "If you continue to say you have a foul odor coming from your body and refuse to take the medication, I will have no choice but to take you to court and get a court order from a judge. That will give the hospital ward the right to give you the medicine and keep you here until you get better." I flopped down on the bed and sat there in disbelief. I could not believe this doctor could have the legal right to give me psychiatric medication for a chemical imbalance I did not have. I was terrified. (By what means would he give me the medication against my will, I thought)

Dr. Walsh left the room and said he would see me on Monday. Over the weekend, I thought about how Dr. Landry could have helped me from the first day I found the book. All she had to do was get the book and talk to the dermatologist. I hated her. Being in the mental ward was not helping me. I could not go to the doctor's office or the library. I was terrified of staying in Chicago anymore because of the threat Dr. Walsh had made about forcing me to stay in the ward. If he felt that way, other doctors might as well. I had to think of a way out of the ward. I wanted to go back to the library and get a telephone number or address from the book *The Human Body Odor* so I could talk to or write to the book's authors. I would tell Dr. Walsh on Monday that if he let me see a dermatologist and the dermatologist said I do not have a body odor; I would start taking medicine. The fact was, I was obsessed with seeing a dermatologist. I knew I had to get out of the hospital to help myself. When I found the book, I found hope for life. I kept telling myself I needed to see a dermatologist. I did not understand why the doctors could not smell the odor, but I knew it was possible from the little information I had read in the book. I had been in the ward for four days and three nights.

On Monday, I woke up at 5:30 a.m. I ate breakfast, showered, and waited for Dr. Walsh to come. Like clockwork, at 7:30 a.m., Dr. Walsh came in.

"Hi, Ms. Wilson," he said. "Did you get some rest this weekend?" "I feel much better," I told him.

He said, "I want you to start on the medication today." "Dr. Walsh," I said, "I do not smell the odor anymore." "Why? What happened?" he asked.

"I just don't," I said. "But I wanted to ask you if it would be possible for me to see a dermatologist. If the dermatologist says I do not have an odor, I will start taking medicine."

"Why do you want to see a dermatologist if you say the odor is gone?" he asked. "I still want to see one, please, Dr. Walsh."

"Okay," he said. "I will try to get a dermatologist up here to see you today." I lay in bed for the rest of the day. I even missed lunch.

At 4:00 p.m., Carol knocked on the door. "Carry, this is Dr. Baldwin. He is a dermatologist, and he needs to see you." I was so excited. Finally, a dermatologist! I sat up on the bed.

"Hi, Carry. What is the problem?" Dr. Baldwin asked, looking at my chart.

I told him, "I have a condition that makes me have a foul body odor. I smell it, and other people I encounter smell it, but doctors keep saying there is no odor."

"Doctors are not other people you encounter?" he asked.

"Of course they are," I said. "But I have a body odor, and they are the ones whom I need to smell the odor."

He cut me off as I told him about the cases in the book. "What do people say you smell like?" he asked.

"A dead rat or garbage," I told him.

"Stand up for me and raise your arms," he said. He smelled my armpits. He did not look down at my shirt, but he pulled the collar back and smelled down my shirt. He asked me, "What do you think you smell like?"

"Like something rotten and garbage."

He asked, "Do you smell the odor right now?"

I said yes. He wrote something down in my chart and stood up. "Have a good day, Ms.

Wilson," he said as he was leaving my room. I followed him; I hadn't yet told him about the case report in the book.

As he left the ward, he handed my chart to Carol behind the front desk. Everything was happening so fast! I called Carol as she put my chart on the chart rack. Another nurse behind the front desk said, "Carry, go sit down."

"I'm not talking to you," I said.

She hollered, "Get away from the counter!"

I told her I was talking to Carol. She told me to stop bringing my ass back and forth to the hospital. I walked back to my room in tears. I told myself that when I cure my body odor, I would make a complaint against that nurse. She had no right to speak to me like that. I felt like a piece of garbage. I cried myself to sleep that night, and I did not eat dinner.

The next morning, Dr. Walsh came to see me earlier than usual. I was eating breakfast.

"Ms. Wilson, I need to speak to you in your room," he said. I sat on my bed. "You saw the dermatologist yesterday?"

"Yes."

"What did he say?"

I stopped breathing for the few seconds it took Dr. Walsh to open my folder and read. "Dr. Baldwin said he did not smell an odor coming from you."

I did not overreact. I used all my strength to hold back the tears. "I want you to start taking the medicine today," he said.

"I told you I do not smell the odor anymore, but I will take a prescription for the medicine home with me just in case the odor comes back," I said calmly.

"I need to see how you react to the medicine," he told me. I saw no way around it; I'd have to take the medicine. I wanted to get out of the hospital. I needed to get to the library and get the information out of the book too.

"Okay, I will take the medicine today," I agreed. "I will tell the nurse," Dr. Walsh said.

I sat there thinking. *What am I going to do?* I knew I couldn't swallow the pill, but I had to act like I was going to. I also knew that when patients take their medicine, they stand in one line, swallow the pill, and open their mouths wide so a nurse can look into their mouths. I didn't know what to do.

Later that day, the nurse said it was time for meds. The nurse handed me a cup of water in one hand and the pill in the other. I took a deep breath and placed the pill on my tongue. I gulped water, and as the water entered my mouth, I spit the pill into the cup. I opened my mouth wide so the nurse could look in. She nodded her head. I was scared she would look in my cup, but she didn't. I waited five minutes and then flushed the pill down the toilet.

The next morning, Dr. Walsh came earlier than usual again. I sat at the breakfast table.

He asked me how I felt.

"Okay," I said.

"How did the medicine make you feel?" he asked.

"Could we go to my room and talk?" I asked him. I did not even think about asking the nurse about the medicine's side effects, so I used the walk to my room to think about what I should say.

"The medication made my head hurt a little," I told him.

He said, "That is a normal side effect. Once your body gets used to the medicine, the headaches will stop. I will discharge you today." I was happy!

Dr. Walsh referred me to Dr. Lauren Smith, a registered nurse (RN) and a psychiatrist. He thought I would like to see her because she could help me with my depression and hygiene issues. "She can see you tomorrow at 11:00 a.m.," he said.

"Thank you so much," I replied. The doctor also gave me a prescription for the crazy pills, a token, and all my belongings. I was discharged at 1:00 p.m. There was enough time for me to get to the library. Immediately after I got off the elevator on the hospital's first floor, I threw the prescription for the crazy pills in a garbage can. I walked extra fast to get to the library. I asked the librarian for some notebook paper and a pen. I found the book in the same row where I found it the first time. I sat down and looked at the book's last page; no address or telephone number existed. I looked at the first page again—nothing. I looked through the book, not reading but scoping for phone numbers or addresses that stood out.

I wrote out facts and symptoms that I could relate to. The library had other books on the condition of bromhidrosis. So, I wrote out different treatment options, including topical solutions, anticholinergic drugs, and surgery. I asked a guy sitting next to me what time it was.

"4:30 p.m.," he said.

I was hungry and disappointed that I had not found an address or telephone number in any of the books I had read. Still, I had gathered enough information to show to the new doctor.

As I put the book back on the shelf, I thought that the new doctor needed to see this book.

She could read the case reports and understand that it was possible for me to have the odor and for some people to smell it and others not to. I had to get this book. God would not be mad if I stole this book and brought it back after I showed it to the doctor.

I opened the book to the first page and tore the front cover off because that was where the sensor was. I put the book in my bag and went to the first floor. Two checkpoint systems were in front of both exits, but I was sure I had torn off the sensor on the book's front cover. I walked through the checkpoint, and the alarm went off. I stood there, looking like the checkpoint system had malfunctioned. A security guard came running from the back of the library. I turned and walked to the library's front desk and tried to look puzzled. The security guard asked me if I had another book from another library.

"Sometimes other books from other medical libraries set off the checkpoint system," he said.

I told him, "Yes, I do."

He asked, "Can I look at it?" I handed him the book, and he turned to the back cover. There it was, "The property of the University of Chicago Health and Science Library on Polk Street."

He looked at me and said, "This book belongs to this library."

I stood there, stuck. I couldn't move, hoping he would not call the cops and put me back in the mental hospital. Dr. Walsh would question why I had tried to steal the book if I thought I did not have the odor. He would know I had lied to him. I was terrified; Dr. Walsh would surely take me to court and have me admitted.

The security guard told me to leave the library and never return. As I ran out of the library, I did not feel bad about trying to steal the book; I felt terrible because I had gotten caught. I did not cry or feel bad as I rode the bus home. I had a lot of essential information to show Dr. Smith. She would understand me better.

I did not sleep well that night. My father did not come by my apartment, so I had to borrow some bus fare from my neighbor, Lewis, to get to my appointment.

I made it to Dr. Smith's office at 10:50 a.m. I knocked on her door.

"Hi, Ms. Wilson, come in and have a seat," she said, opening the door and pointing towards a chair. I sat down and looked around her office. It was not like a regular examination room with medical supplies. There was a couch, a bookshelf with many books, and a comfortable chair that I sat in. There was a little refrigerator, and her desk was big and covered with pictures of kids. The room had a warm and comfortable feel.

Dr. Smith had a folder in her hand that she was looking at. She said, "Let me start by saying you walked past me when you entered the door, and I did not smell you. My friends always ask me to smell things because I have a nose like a wolf, and if you smelled foul, I would tell you, "she said.

I got up and thanked her for seeing me. "Ms. Wilson, are you leaving?" she asked.

"Yes! I am," I told her.

"Please come back in, and we can discuss the odor," she said. But she had said she did not smell me within the first five minutes of meeting me. There was nothing I could say to change her mind. I did not enjoy talking to a psychiatrist, anyway.

"I am sorry for wasting your time," I told her. People are not as open to telling you the truth if you smell bad. They will talk behind your back and make indirect comments about your body odor. This is a fact; I have lived it.

When I returned home, I had two options: stay in Chicago and try to convince doctors that I had body odor or move to New Orleans and see new doctors. Over the next week, I talked to my father and sister about moving to New Orleans. My father did not want me to go, but he knew I had to do it. I waited a week for my father tuo get paid so he could buy me a bus ticket. If my family were in New York, I would have moved there, but my family was in New Orleans.

The health care was horrible, and living below the poverty line was normal. I did not know this when I decided to move to New Orleans to get help; I would discover this was the worst move of my life.

THE MOVE

In 1998, my father bought me a one-way bus ticket to New Orleans and gave me one-hundred dollars. The bus ride was long. My sister knew I was coming but thought I was only going to stay for two weeks. I planned to find a dermatologist to diagnose me with bromhidrosis and surgically remove my sweat glands.

Once I made it to New Orleans, I called and asked my sister to pick me up from the bus station and to bring Sherry. I could not wait to see my daughter. When my sister saw how many suitcases I had, she said, "For someone who isn't staying long, you brought a lot of clothes."

She introduced me to her boyfriend, who put my suitcases in the back of the truck. He seemed like a nice guy. We got in the car. Sherry kept hugging me; she was so glad I was there. I was happy to see my daughter.

"You don't know how long you'll be here?" she asked. "Until I get the help I need," I replied.

"What you got? An odor?" my sister asked.

I leaned into the truck's front seat and hit her on the arm, nodding toward her boyfriend. "Don't say that in front of him," I whispered.

"Girl, we are family. Daddy said your ass is going crazy," she told me.

I did not know my father had told my sister about my

medical condition. I did not care, but I did not appreciate him telling her I was crazy.

"You must stay at Mama's house because I don't have enough room," my sister said. "I'll stay with Mama," I agreed. I had not seen my mother in three years.

When we made it to my mother's house, I was pleasantly surprised by my mother's beauty. I was glad to see her. My mother, sister, and I talked well into the night, but I had bigger business to take care of. I asked my mother if I could stay with her for a while.

"Sure," she replied.

I also asked her for the name of the free hospital in New Orleans. "Charity Hospital," she replied.

I asked her to please write down the address of the local welfare office. I knew I would need to get on welfare (public assistance) to have bus fare to get around New Orleans.

As my sister and Sherry left for the night, my sister told me I needed to take back custody of Sherry soon. I pleaded with her to give me time to find a job first.

On my second day in New Orleans, I applied for welfare for Sherry and me. I got a dermatology appointment with Dr. Hogan at the Charity Dermatology Clinic in December of 1998. It was October 1998, so I had to wait two months for my appointment. I gave my mother some money for the rent and bought some food for the house once I was approved for welfare. My sister kept pressuring me to take back custody of Sherry, so I had no choice but to get my daughter back.

My two brothers, my stepfather, my mother, and now me and my daughter were all living at my mother's house; it was just as overcrowded as my sister's apartment. I begged my sister to talk to our cousin Tammy about letting Sherry and me stay with her until I could afford an apartment. My cousin had a two-bedroom apartment that she lived in by herself. My sister talked Tammy into letting Sherry and I move in with her, but my sister informed me that Tammy said, "Your ass must get a job and help pay the rent." I had not come to New Orleans to get a job; I had come to find a cure, but I could not stay with anyone for free, not even family. I knew it was a bad idea, but I needed a place to stay, and staying with my cousin would put my daughter within walking distance of the local school while also providing me with a room.

I called my cousin and thanked her for letting me and Sherry stay with her. I assured my cousin I would get a job as soon as possible.

Sherry and I moved in with my cousin immediately. Once we all settled into our rooms, Tammy called me into her room. "Carry, you have got to get a job, and I do not want to hear anything about you smelling bad. I have been around you twice and do not smell you." She said she never wanted to talk about my smell. I agreed.

I got a job at a gas station as a cashier in late October. My coworkers wasted no time in remarking that something stunk, or they'd cough whenever I was around. They also said their heads hurt. I was used to different verbal reactions, but people saying their head hurt was something new.

A couple of months after moving to New Orleans, I suddenly started having these minor episodes that I thought were a type of nervous attacks. I usually just took deep breaths and drank a cup of water, and I could calm myself down. Whenever someone came close to me, I would become extremely nervous and start sweating. I remember when my supervisor was training me on the register at the gas station and showing me how to take an inventory of the store's products. She saw that I was physically uncomfortable. She told me to calm down and relax.

The good and bad thing about this job was that I worked alone during my shift. My only contact with my coworkers was when we changed shifts, which only took twenty minutes.

My appointment with the dermatologist was approaching; it was less than a week away. I was feeling uncomfortable at work. I hated those twenty minutes it took to change shifts. My coworkers always commented about my body odor during the shift change. I was not making much money at the gas station, although it allowed me to make enough to pay my cousin one hundred dollars a month in rent.

Finally, the day of my appointment with the dermatologist arrived. I was up early to get to my 10:00 a.m. appointment. I had all the information I had gathered on bromhidrosis to show Dr. Hogan. I arrived at the clinic and filled out the new patient forms. The waiting room was overflowing with people. I waited two hours before Dr. Hogan called me into the examination room. I watched her facial expressions as she read the patient forms I had filled out.

"Okay, Ms. Wilson, so you think you have bromhidrosis? Raise your arms." She smelled under my arms and down my shirt. "With whom do you live?" she asked.

"My cousin," I replied.

"What does your cousin say you smell like?" she asked.

"My cousin said she does not smell me. We do not talk about my body odor." I told her I had gotten all this information from published medical books related to this condition. I asked her whether she had ever heard of this condition. She said she had little knowledge about the condition but was sure I did not have it.

Dr. Hogan said, "This condition is rare; you do not have it."

Once again, I tried and failed to convince doctors that I could have it, although it was a rare condition. People saying they did not smell the foul odor I had coming from my body was a symptom of the condition. Doctors treated me like there was no way I could have this rare condition, but by those standards, my condition would be rare. Dr. Hogan even said I had a better chance of winning the lottery than I did of having this condition.

"You do not have this condition, and I do not smell you," she repeated. I asked her to look at the case reports I gave her. I pointed out the specific case report of the girl with a foul body odor that some people smelled and others did not. I continued explaining that the dermatologist did not smell the patient's odor but still helped her with other testing methods. Dr. Hogan sorted through the case report.

"I do not see that case report you are speaking of," she said. I realize I'd left it at home.

She asked me what kind of soap I used. I told her and explained that the soap and water do not stop my body odor. I started crying.

"You are crying," she said. "Are you depressed?"

I said no. If I had answered yes, she would say I needed to see a psychiatrist. I thanked her for seeing me and asked if I could see another dermatologist.

"Sure. Just make another appointment at the front desk," she said.

I made another appointment in the same clinic to see another dermatologist. When I returned home that night, I fell into a deep depression, and I started missing work, which caused problems between my cousin and me. She had no idea what it was like to stink like shit and have no one believe you. The more I saw doctors, the worse I felt, but I had to keep seeing doctors to get cured. I had to make it through the feeling of hopelessness, or I would have to go back into the mental ward.

In late December of 1998, they fired me from the gas station, and my cousin told me to get another job or move out. I called my mother and begged her to talk to her boss at the nursing home to see if she could get me a job as a housekeeper. I also begged my sister to let my daughter move back in with her until I could find another job. I told her there was too much tension between Tammy and me. My sister reluctantly agreed to let my daughter move back in with her. My sister's boyfriend thought I was taking advantage of her because he did not smell an odor from me on the day they picked me up from the bus station. He thought I did not want to raise my daughter. I asked my sister not to tell her boyfriend about my business. I assured her I would try to get a job with our mother at the nursing home.

Later that night, I informed my cousin that I would apply for a job at the nursing home where my mother worked.

"Whatever," she said.

The following day, my mother called and told me to come to her workplace before noon and ask to speak to a lady named Ms. Hattie about the housekeeping position. I immediately got dressed and caught the bus to my mother's job.

Once I arrived, I informed the receptionist that I needed to speak with Ms. Hattie in housekeeping. Ms. Hattie approached me.

"Hello, you must be Carry; you look just like your mother," she said.

She asked me a few questions about my work history and handed me an application to fill out. I gave the completed application back to her.

"I see here you have two years of housekeeping experience," she asked. "Yes, I do," I replied.

"I need some housekeepers right now, and your mother is one of my best workers," she

said.

"It runs in the family," I replied.

She told me she would review my application and call me

before 4:00 p.m. I thanked her for interviewing me and went down the hall looking for my mother.

Her coworker told me, "Your mother is on her lunch break at a restaurant down the street. She should be back in thirty minutes." I went outside and waited for her to return from her lunch break.

I stood in front of the nursing home talking to one of the elderly residents. She was so happy I was talking to her, and I did not mind. It made me feel good to make someone else happy.

As I waited for my mother to return from lunch, I saw a guy walking toward me. The closer he got, the more familiar he looked. He looked like Corey, someone I'd had a summer fling with when I visited my mother and sister once in New Orleans. We had been hot and heavy until the end of that summer. He had cried and begged me to stay in New Orleans. We had fun hanging out during the summer, but I told him I was going home. I promised to stay in touch with him when I returned to Chicago but I never called or wrote to him. The guy walking toward me looked like him. When he got close enough, I recognized it was him. I was not sure how to react. If I hugged him, he would smell me. He walked right up to me and hugged me tightly.

"Hey, Corey! How did you know I was here?" I asked.

"I saw your brother, and he was not sure where you were living, and he suggested I come by your mom's job to ask about you," he said.

I became extremely nervous and started sweating. The odor became more intense. I could smell my deodorant, the baby powder, and body odor mixing into one scent. It smelled like funk and mildew, but he stood beside me, smiling and talking as if he didn't smell anything.

"Do you want to get something to eat later?" he asked.

“Sure,” I said. I gave him my cousin’s address and phone number and told him to pick me up that night at 7:00 p.m.

When I got home, Ms. Hattie had not called me about the job, so I called her. “Hi, Ms. Hattie, this is Carry Wilson,” I said.

“I was going to call you,” she told me. “I want you to start tomorrow morning. Be here at 8:00 a.m.”

I told her, “I will see you tomorrow.”

When my cousin came home, I started getting ready for my date. I told her I had a nursing home job starting the next day.

“Good. You can pay me the back rent you owe me,” she responded. “I will pay you with my first check,” I agreed.

I was happy to get some of the tension out of the house. My cousin noticed me getting dressed.

“Where are you going?” she asked. “Out with a friend.”

“A guy friend?” “Yeah,” I replied.

“But you have a body odor,” she pointed out.

“Girl, please, just because I am going out with a guy does not mean I do not have a body odor,” I said. “I am a woman just like you. I want to be loved, too.”

She went into her room and closed the door.

Corey arrived at 7:00 p.m. I went downstairs, and he met me on the porch, hugged me tightly, and said I looked nice. As we sat in his car, he said he needed to wash the inside of his car because it smelled like shit.

“It does not smell like shit to me,” I said.

At dinner, Corey told me he had never stopped thinking about me after I left and that he had missed me. He said I was his first love.

After dinner, it was clear Corey wanted to have sex. It felt good for a guy to show any interest in me. I felt so ugly because I smelled so bad. That night, I did not care about the odor if he did not care. Having any man spend time with me made me feel like a regular woman, even if he only wanted sex.

Being intimate with Corey felt good. He gave me a part of my life back that night. I fell in love with the idea that if Corey (or any man) wanted me, I was normal, even if I smelled bad. The thought that he would accept me with my body odor made me feel good, but the fact was that no man accepting me with my body odor would complete me or make me normal. I had to be happy within myself; I was not happy because I had a body odor. I did not want to smell bad.

Corey dropped me off at home early in the morning. He did not give me a telephone number or tell me the next time he would call me before he drove off.

I took a good shower and got to work at 8:00 a.m. They gave me a sheet of paper with my job description; it assigned me to four hallways. I had to mop and sweep all the hallways, which were ten feet long. I also had to wipe down the furniture in ten rooms.

After working three hours, I was hot from all the bending down, moving furniture, sweeping, and mopping back and forth. My body odor was unbearable. I smelled like a dead rat, and all I could think about was that my mother worked there and I would embarrass her.

At 11:30 a.m., Ms. Hattie entered the hall and told me to take a thirty-minute lunch break. I went to the employee break room. I sat at a table with two female employees and a guy. I ate a bag of chips for lunch.

As I left the break room to return to work, the two women sitting at the table with me started laughing. I did not think they were laughing at me, but it bothered me that they laughed after I got up.

I returned to my hall and started cleaning the rooms and hallways. I was in a room, bent down behind a chair, wiping it down, when I heard a woman say, "Whoever is cleaning this hall needs to change the mop water. It stinks like a dirty mop." I ran to the door and looked down the hallway; it was one of the women from the break room.

"What did you say?" I asked.

She replied, "Your mop water is dirty; you don't smell the stench of mildew?" "Okay, I will change the water," I replied.

After work, I stopped by my sister's house to see my daughter. I told Candice I was working, and she asked, "For how long, and did anybody smell you? You are going to quit."

"Are you telling me you do not smell an odor from me?" I asked.

"Carry, your body is changing from a little girl to a woman's. It is a hygiene problem, not a medical problem."

"Do you smell me?" I asked.

"You smell musty sometimes, but I think it's normal. It's not as serious as you are making it out to be," she replied. I respect my sister so much. She was the only person who was there for me through this entire ordeal, but the fact was, this was my life, and it was important.

"I will keep the job because I want to leave Tammy's house. I don't think things will work out with me living there," I told her.

My sister said Tammy had lived with another cousin, and things had ended badly between them. Because of that situation, Tammy was stern about her house rules and rent.

"Whatever, I have to get out of there soon and give her back her privacy," I said. I gave my sister my food stamp card and told her to buy groceries for her house since Sherry was staying there.

"Come over for Christmas," she said. I accepted.

I did not see my cousin that night before I went to bed, but I saw her in the morning while I was getting ready for work.

"That's right, go to work," she said. She asked me for my food stamp card. I told her, "Candice has it right now."

"Why does Candice have your food stamp card? You stay

here," she said in a thunderous voice.

"But Sherry stays over there. I had to give her something to let Sherry stay there." "You already owe me two months' rent, and you gave away all your food stamps,"

Tammy said.

"I did not give them all away. I will get the food stamp card back tonight," I told her.

My cousin was right, but I did not want my sister to give my daughter back to me yet. I left the house in tears. I had to return to this job and embarrass my mother with this body odor, and my cousin was on me for rent money. My stomach turned as the bus approached the nursing home. I felt nervous and sweaty. Before getting to the nursing home, I got off the bus down the street because I knew I was not going in. After that lady had said my mop water smelled like mildew, I could not face my coworkers.

I got on another bus and went to my sister's house. I knocked on my sister's door. When she opened the door and saw me standing there, she yelled, "You quit! Tammy is going to throw your ass out of her house, and what about Sherry?"

I told her I needed to make another appointment to see a dermatologist after Christmas. I had also considered putting Sherry in foster care until I was cured.

"I know you cannot care for her, and your boyfriend does not want her here," I said.

"That is not true. My man wants you to get your life together and be a mother to your child," she told me.

I started crying. "You think I enjoy living like this? Why do I have to have body odor? Why won't doctors investigate what I am saying? I told them to get the book, but they wouldn't even try."

"Have you tried to get the book down here?" she asked.

"No, but I will. I cannot keep moving Sherry back and forth. Until I get cured, I need to place her somewhere."

"You are serious about putting her in foster care?" my sister asked. "Yes, I am," I said.

I used my sister's phone and called every medical library I could find in the Yellow Pages. None of the libraries had the book *The Human Body Odor*. My search produced nothing.

I asked my sister for the food stamp card.

"Why? There are no more food stamps on it," she replied. "You spent them all?" I asked.

"Carry, I have five mouths to feed, including Sherry," she told me. "I can keep her for three more weeks, but you must make a move. Decide what you will do at that point."

Putting Sherry in foster care was a good, bad, and scary idea. I knew I had to give my cousin some money for rent, or we would have a big argument about those food stamps. I went home at 10:30 p.m. I hoped my cousin was fast asleep, as she usually was. I had a key, so I opened the door slowly. I tip-toed through the house and reached my room across from Tammy's. I could hear my cousin getting out of bed as I put my purse on the bed. She came out of her room.

"Your mother called and spoke with me; she said you did not go to work today." "I did not like that job. I am going to get another one," I replied.

"You must be kidding me. Do you have your food stamp card?" Tammy asked. "Candace spent them all," I replied.

Tammy walked out, went into her room, and closed the door. I waited five minutes and then knocked on her door. "I am sorry. I know I owe you money. I will move out as soon as possible," I told her. She did not respond. I knew I could not stay with anyone for free. I needed a family member to help me and let me stay with them for free, and I would give them monetarily what I could until I was cured of my body odor. This was my ordeal, and my cousin had bills to pay. Being there added to her bills.

I sat on the bed, thinking: *Where am I going to live? In a shelter?*

The phone rang. My cousin hollered, "Get the phone!"

It was Corey. "Can I come and get you tonight?" he asked. "Only if we can stay the whole night in a hotel," I told him. "Okay, I am on my way now," he said.

I packed up all my clothes; I would move out that night. I would take one big bag with me to a shelter and store the other suitcase and bags at my sister's apartment.

Corey arrived, and as I left the apartment, I handed my cousin her key and told her again how sorry I was about everything not working out between us, but she was so mad that she did not acknowledge me. It was okay. I still loved and appreciated her, and we would mend our relationship later.

I was sweating profusely from dragging two suitcases and a big bag towards Corey's car. I asked him to take me to my sister's house so I could drop off my suitcases. He asked why I was carrying suitcases. I told him I had to move out of my cousin's apartment, and he looked concerned and asked me, "Are you moving out tonight?"

"Yes, tonight," I said.

He asked me where I was going to live.

I hollered, "I don't know where I will live!"

He asked me again, "Where are you going to live?"

I warned him not to ask me again. "I will probably go to a shelter," I replied. "You would go to a shelter?" he asked.

"Yes, I will go to a shelter," I retorted.

My sister was standing on her porch when Corey and I pulled up and got out of the car. "Tammy kicked your ass out?" she asked.

"No," I said, "but I decided it was best to move out tonight."

"Mama called and said Ms. Hattie fired you. Ms. Hattie was mad you filled out all that paperwork for nothing," she said. My sister said I could stay with her for a week. She informed me she and her man were having personal problems and arguing a lot, so this was not a good time for me to stay with them for longer.

"Okay," I replied.

She looked at Corey and asked me, "Is that the boy you used to talk to when you were here last time?"

"Yes," I said.

"How did you find him?" she asked.

"I didn't. He found me at Mama's job."

She whispered in my ear, "You had sex with him?"

"Yeah, I did," I answered.

"But you have a body odor that bothers you so much."

"I will see you in the morning," I said, walking away from her and getting into the car. I would not stand there and explain myself to her. I was a woman just like her, and I had needs and feelings, too.

Corey and I spent the night in the hotel, and I fell in love with him because he was with me even though I smelled bad, and he did not care. Corey never said directly to my face that I smelled bad, but he commented about something smelling bad, just like my coworkers and people back home. I often acted like I did not hear him.

When Corey dropped me off at my sister's house the next day, I asked him to give me his phone number. He gave me his beeper number.

I walked into my sister's house, and she and her boyfriend were arguing. They did not see me enter, so I stepped back out the door and sat on the porch. After twenty minutes, my sister's boyfriend came storming out the door. I said hello, but he did not hear me. He jumped in his car and drove off. My sister came out the door behind him.

"Carry, I did not know you were out here," she said.

"Are you and your boyfriend arguing because you said I could stay here?" I asked. "We have been on the verge of breaking up for a while," she told me. "He's not coming back. We will work out our problems." She said she had to finish Christmas shopping, and for the first time that day, I realized it was Christmas Eve.

At 10:30 a.m., my sister asked me if I wanted to go shopping. "No, I just want to chill out for the day," I said. But really, I wanted to be alone and cry. No matter how much I tried not to cry about my life, I could not help it. I did not want to live in New Orleans; I did not want to smell bad. I just wanted a normal life. I prayed to God, "Please help me and make this odor disappear."

There was no one else in the house. My sister was out shopping. I cried myself to sleep and awoke to many little knocks on the door. It was Sherry with my nieces and nephew. Sherry hugged me tightly.

"Mama, are you staying here?" she asked.

"Yes!" I replied. The kids were happy to see me, but when I looked at my daughter, all I saw was pain. I had moved her to New Orleans and did not spend enough time with her. My sister could not take care of my daughter and her own kids.

I went into the kitchen and made the kids dinner. My daughter was overjoyed because I was acting like a mother. While I cooked, she hung around the kitchen and looked at me. She came and hugged me around the waist, and this unsettled me as I thought about putting her in foster care.

My sister came in late that night, and she and I sat on the front porch well into the early morning, talking about our childhood growing up in Chicago. It was refreshing to talk about memories when I did not have this foul odor coming from my body. My sister told me she bought Sherry two toys for

Christmas.

The next morning, we all awoke to music and my sister hollering, "Get up! It is Christmas. Come on, Merry Christmas!" We all ran into the front room, where their toys sat under the tree. The kids opened their toys and screamed with excitement. My sister gave Sherry a doll and a board game. I was happy my sister brought my daughter presents. Christmas was different that year. I had this odor and could not afford to buy Sherry the Christmas gifts she wanted. Sherry and I were so grateful to my sister.

I waited until after the New Year's holiday to make a doctor's appointment and call a foster care agency. The first business day after New Year's, I looked through the Yellow Pages and found a dermatologist, Dr. Kastle. I got an appointment with him two weeks later, which gave me time to look for a job and place Sherry in a foster home.

I called an organization that mentioned foster care in the Yellow Pages. A woman answered the phone.

"Hi, my name is Carry Wilson, and I have a seven-year-old daughter I cannot properly provide for," I said. I told her I was poor and I was taking my daughter from house to house. I wanted to put my daughter in foster care until I could get a stable job and a place for us to live. The woman informed me that people could not just put their children in foster care. She said that was not how it worked. She continued to tell me that children are placed in foster care when they are put up for adoption or removed from their homes. "Do you want to put your daughter up for adoption?" she asked.

"No, but I cannot properly take care for my daughter. I have nervous breakdowns every other day, which is not good for her."

"Where do you live now?" she asked.

"I live with my sister but must move as soon as possible."

"Can your sister let your daughter live with her temporarily?" she asked. "No. My sister is struggling, taking care of her own children," I replied. "You do not have any family members your child can stay with?"

"I have no one," I told her.

"What is your sister's address and telephone number?" she asked. She said someone would call me back soon. I hung up the phone and just sat there. I did not know it would be so hard to place Sherry in foster care, but I considered putting her up for adoption. My life was on hold until I could be cured.

The phone rang; it was Corey. "Have you found somewhere to live yet?" he asked. "No," I replied.

"My friend told me his ex-girlfriend has a two-bedroom apartment and needs a roommate. You have one child and are looking for a place to stay. Her name is Lisa. Get a piece of paper and write down her number. Lisa is expecting a call from you today."

I felt overwhelmed with love for Corey; he must love my daughter and me. Why would he put so much effort into helping me find somewhere for us to live? He told me to call Lisa right then and that he would call me later.

As I called Lisa, my sister Candice and her best friend Linda entered the house. I felt uncomfortable around Linda sometimes because of the odor. Linda had no idea the strange odor she complained about when she was around me was coming from me.

One day, when she came by my sister's house, I sat in the front room, and Linda told my sister she needed to take the garbage can out of the front room because it smelled. My sister said there was no garbage can in the front room. "Carry, she was not talking about you!" my sister exclaimed. I knew it was me.

I liked Linda; she made me feel like a regular home girl, and I appreciated how she talked for hours about men and Chicago with me. However, I did not have the time to speak to her or my sister that day. I told them to get out so I could make a phone call.

I called Lisa. "Hi, my name is Carry. This is Corey's friend." I said.

"I am glad you called. You have one child, a daughter, right?" she asked. "Yes," I replied.

"What is her name?"

"Sherry. She is six years old."

Lisa asked me if I had a job. I told her I had just moved to New Orleans and had not found a decent job, but I was searching.

"I do not do drugs or run a whorehouse," she said.

"Good. I do not do drugs and only have one guy friend," I replied. "When can I meet you and your daughter?" she asked.

"What about tomorrow at 1:00 p.m.?

"That sounds like a good idea. If our meeting goes well tomorrow, as long as you can give me one hundred dollars a month and put some food in the refrigerator until you get a job, we will get along well," she replied.

I got her address and told her, "I will see you tomorrow."

I hung up the phone and went and sat outside with my sister and Linda. They were listening to music. I always had fun just chilling with my sister and Linda.

The next day, I kept Sherry home from school. I combed Sherry's hair and put her in the best-looking outfit borrowed from my niece's clothes. I decided not to put on baby powder, just a little deodorant. I did not want my body odor to be why she did not give me the room.

I made it to Lisa's house at 12:45 p.m. I knocked on the door. She opened the door. "Hi, Carry," she said.

"Hi, Lisa," I answered.

"Is this Sherry?" she asked as she picked Sherry up and nodded for me to come into the house. I walked into the apartment and looked around; it was nice and clean. The kitchen and bathroom were decent. She showed me my room, and I told her I would not give her any problems if she rented me the room. Lisa asked me many questions, trying to get to know me better, and she had a sweet, inviting attitude. She gave Sherry cookies and milk, sat her at the kitchen table, and suggested we talk in the front room.

Lisa asked, "So, when do you want to move in?"

"In two weeks, once I get my welfare check," I told her.

"You can move in before then; as long as you get your check, you give me rent money and food stamps. Please begin looking for work immediately," she said.

"Okay," I said.

She asked me if I had anyone to help me move my furniture. "Like what?" I asked. "Your bed and dressers," she said.

"I just moved here," I told her. "All I have is clothes." "You and your daughter will sleep on the floor?" she asked.

"Yeah," I said. I guess she was not from the ghetto because sleeping on the floor in a house is better than not having anywhere to sleep. I told her, "I am going to get a bed."

She looked at me with doubt, hoping she was not making a mistake in letting me move in with her. She told me I could move in the next day.

When I left her house, I thanked God for Lisa; she was so lovely, and I needed the help.

On my way to my sister's house, I stopped at the store and bought two packs of incense with my last three dollars. I knew I would burn them in my room.

When I got to my sister's house; I told her I was moving in with this girl Corey knew, and her name was Lisa.

"Girl, your ass is crazy. This girl could be a killer," my sister said.

"No, she needs a roommate. She is sweet, and her house is clean," I told her.

I called Corey and asked him to pick me up the next day at

noon so I could move in with Lisa. I told him I loved him, and he said okay. Corey never said he loved me back whenever I told him I loved him. I packed up all of mine and Sherry's clothes that night.

The next morning, at 9:00 a.m., while my sister, Sherry, and I sat in the kitchen eating breakfast, someone knocked on the door. My sister went and answered the door. She returned to the kitchen with her hands over her mouth and looked big-eyed.

"What's wrong? Who is it?" I asked.

"Sherry, go into the back room and be quiet until I come and get you," my sister said. "What's wrong?" I asked.

"Two women from the department of children and welfare office want to see you," she told me. I was confused. I took a deep breath and went to the door.

One woman said, "May we come in?" One sat down as they walked into the house, while the other looked around./.

The woman sitting /said, "My name is Ms. Washington, and I am a child welfare worker. Did you call and report that you could not care for your daughter and were taking her from house to house?"

"Yes, I did," I said. "But I have found somewhere to live now."

Ms. Washington asked me some personal questions and gave me a card with a name and telephone number. She told me to call the number on the card if I became homeless again or needed food help. I said thank you and let them out.

My sister looked out the window blinds and said, "Bitch, you better give up on this odor shit and get a job!"

"This odor is taking over my life. I must get cured!" I cried.

At 11:30 a.m., Corey came, picked up me and Sherry, and dropped us off at our new home at Lisa's.

I knocked on the door, and a guy opened the door and said, "Hi, Carry. I am Barry, Lisa's boyfriend. She is not here right now. She is buying you some sheets and pillows for your bed at the store."

"Oh, I told her I don't have a bed right now," I replied.

He said her grandmother gave her a bed for Sherry and I. I walked into my room, dropped my bags, and started crying. There was a bed and a TV in the room; they hadn't been there the day before.

"Why are you crying?" Barry asked.

"She didn't have to buy all of this," I said.

"Don't cry. Lisa is always helping people," Barry told me.

Corey put my suitcases in my room and told me he would talk to me later. I closed my door. I lit some incense, opened the window, and put a towel at the bottom of the door. I would not stink up this girl's house.

When Lisa returned, she asked me, "What is that smell in your room?" I told her I had lit some incense. I thanked her for the bed, TV, and pillows. "Thank you so much," I told her.

"My boyfriend told me you were crying. I know your situation, and I do not mind helping you," she said.

As I asked her what she had been told about my situation, her boyfriend called her, and she asked Sherry, "What did you eat today?"

Sherry said, "Nothing."

Lisa said, "Carry, don't act shy. You can cook you and your daughter something to eat whenever you want to, okay?" I fried some chicken and made rice for dinner.

Later that night, after Sherry fell asleep, I knocked on Lisa's bedroom door and asked her if she had to work the next day.

She yelled through the door, "Yes, I have to work, but my boyfriend will be here." As I walked away from her door, Lisa came, stuck her head out the door, and asked me, "When do you think you will start looking for a job?"

I asked her if I could speak with her in the front room.

"Sure," she said.

We went and sat on the couch. I told her, "I will be frank with you. I have an exceedingly rare medical condition, but it has been hard for me to get diagnosed and treated by doctors. Until I get cured, I must put my daughter up for adoption."

"Carry, no!" she said. "Please do not put your daughter up for adoption."

"I have no choice," I told her. "It will be easier for me to see doctors and get cured." She frowned. "What type of condition do you have?"

I told her to wait one moment, and I got up, went to my room, got the information on bromhidrosis, and gave it to her.

She read a couple of lines and said, "You have a body odor?" "Yes, but it's a medical condition."

"Why don't I smell you?" she asked.

"Remember when you came into my room today and asked about the smell? You were smelling my body odor and the incense mixing and making a funky smell."

"But it was not a funky smell," she said. "I did not like the smell of that incense."

"Well, most people smell me, but some do not."

She looked genuinely concerned and told me not to give my daughter up for adoption. I reassured her I would look for a job soon, but I needed to call some adoption agencies the next day.

"How is Sherry getting to school tomorrow?" she asked. "She is not going. I am serious about the adoption." "Please, think of other options," she said.

"I will," I told her.

The bed was comfortable, and the covers were so warm.]'

|It was the most comfortable, restful, and peaceful sleep I had experienced since my body odor had begun.

The next morning, I woke up at 8:00 a.m. I looked through the Yellow Pages. I found an adoption agency, and as I reached for the phone, it rang; it was Lisa.

"Please tell me you have not called an adoption agency," she said.

I told her I was about to. She told me an old friend of her grandmother was a legally registered foster parent. She had discussed my situation with her grandmother, who called her friend, Ms. Tyler. Ms. Tyler already had four other foster kids, all girls. Lisa informed me that her grandmother wanted me to know that once a child was in the welfare system, it would not be easy for me to regain custody of my daughter.

"If you feel comfortable letting Sherry live with Ms. Tyler, you can see Sherry and talk to her whenever you want. You and Ms. Tyler can establish a temporary guardianship agreement," she said. Lisa asked me if I wanted Ms. Tyler to call me.

"Yes, I want to speak with her," I said.

Later that day, Ms. Tyler called me. "Hi, my name is Betty Tyler, and you have a seven-year-old daughter you want to put up for adoption? I hope you understand after talking with Lisa that you cannot just place your child in foster care, and putting your child up for adoption may not be your best or only option."

"I know," I said. "I cannot just place my daughter in foster care, and adoption was my only recourse until Lisa told me about you," I replied.

"Well, I am sure Lisa told you a little about me. I would be more than happy to come over and meet you and your daughter. You and Sherry can come by my house, look around, and we can get to know each other."

"I can come over today," I replied. I was not worried about letting Sherry go live with Ms. Tyler. Lisa was a genuinely nice person, and I trusted her judgment. Ms. Tyler was a legally registered foster parent, but I still needed to meet her to see what she was like in person.

When Ms. Tyler arrived, I opened the door and said hello as

I looked her up and down.

She was a well-dressed older woman. She showed me some pictures of her home and foster daughters. I felt amazingly comfortable with her. She asked Sherry to sit by her, and asked her about school and how old she was.

Ms. Tyler asked me when I wanted Sherry to move in with her. I said as soon as possible.

She asked if Sherry and I would like to see her home, and I said yes. On the way to her home, she stopped at a fast-food restaurant and bought something for Sherry and me to eat.

When we got to her house, it was beautiful inside and out. She showed me the room Sherry would sleep in, which was nice.

Over the next week, I explained to Sherry that she would move in with Ms. Tyler until I could get us somewhere to stay. Sherry started crying. She did not want to go to live with Ms.

Tyler. I explained that she would be okay, and I would call her every day and visit her sometimes.

Ms. Tyler and I had to go to a notary public so I could sign over guardianship to her. This would allow her to enroll Sherry in a school near her home.

After Sherry moved in with Ms. Tyler, I put into action all those years of my father teaching me how to get a job before the in-person interview. I called fast food restaurants and asked to speak to the hiring manager or supervisor of the restaurant. I would say, "Hi, my name is Carry Wilson. I filled out an application and checked your hiring status."

I would get an interview, and the interviewer would say, "I couldn't find your application, so you need to fill out another one."

I would get jobs repeatedly by calling and saying this. I told Lisa I got the job, and she was happy. I told her I would give her a little more rent, but I also wanted to save some money to get an apartment to get Sherry back.

On my first day of work, not even one hour into my shift, one of my coworkers walked past me and said, "Something stinks." I went to the bathroom and cried. I calmed down, took a deep breath, and returned to work. After working four hours, my supervisor told me to punch out for a thirty-minute lunch break. I left for my lunch break, quit, and never returned.

When Lisa asked me how my first day of work went, I told her it was good. I knew I had to get a newspaper, look in the hiring section, and get another job. A hotel was hiring housekeepers.

I went the next morning and filled out the application. When I turned the application back in at the front desk, I asked the clerk for the name of the housekeeping supervisor and a hotel business card.

She said, "Ms. Gray is the housekeeping supervisor." I left the hotel and went to the first payphone I saw.

I called the hotel and put on my best white voice. "Hi, may I speak to Ms. Gray?" The clerk said, "I will switch you right now."

When Ms. Gray came on the phone, I said, "Ms. Gray, my name is Carry Wilson, and I just filled out an application. I want to be a housekeeper, and I have hotel housekeeping experience. I would love to work for this hotel."

Ms. Gray told me to come in the next morning at 8:00 a.m. for an interview.

The next morning, she interviewed me and hired me. I started that morning after I filled out all the paperwork. Lisa never knew I had stopped working.

For the next two months, I worked at the hotel. I worked alone, and the way the hotel was built, there was no inside hallway. I entered the hotel rooms from an outside balcony, so I did not have to worry about stinking up a hallway.

At 5:00 a.m., I started my work shifts, so by the time the

other housekeepers came in to start their shifts, I was halfway through my work shift, so my contact with my coworkers was minimal. I was working and concentrating on getting my apartment.

Sherry was in school and thriving. I spoke with her often. I would see Corey at least once a week. My life had some normalcy for a while. But one morning, I got up for work, and while in the shower, I noticed my menstrual cycle had begun. I hated how heavily I bled during the five days of my cycle.

I got to work at 5:00 a.m. It was a warm, humid day, and my body odor was overpowering with my menstrual cycle and the warm weather. I cleaned six rooms before 8:00

a.m. That week, the hotel had contracted with a trucking company, so I had to clean specific rooms first because the truck drivers always came early. Two truck drivers arrived and entered two rooms I had cleaned earlier. Five minutes later, one of them came out of the room and said, "This room stinks," as he headed for the front desk. My supervisor approached me twenty minutes later and said, "Carry, you need to wash your mop out. Two guests complained that their rooms smelled 'stale and funky.' This was not the first time someone compared my odor to a dirty mop.

I left work in tears, but I could not quit. I had to get my apartment and get Sherry back; she wanted to be with me.

I had another appointment with Dr. Kastle the next day. I called my job and told them I had to take the next day off and I would bring a doctor's note, but my supervisor told me I did not need to bring a doctor's note; I should take care of my business for the day and get back to work. I was an excellent worker at every job I had, and I was valuable.

I got to Dr. Kastle's office at 9:30 a.m. I filled out the new patient forms and asked the nurse to make a copy of the information I had brought on bromhidrosis and put it in my chart.

The nurse escorted me to an examination room.

Dr. Kastle came in and said, “Hi, Ms. Wilson. I see here you think you have bromhidrosis.” I noticed he could not pronounce the condition either. He asked me if he was the only doctor I had seen about this body odor. I said no.

“What did the other doctors say?” he asked.

“They said they did not smell an odor coming from me,” I answered. “The nurse will bring you a gown,” he said.

The nurse told me to get undressed and put the gown on. The nurse and Dr. Kastle returned to the room once I put on the gown. Dr. Kastle told me to lie on the table and stretch out my arms. He sniffed closely at my armpits and up and down my body. He sniffed my vagina. He wrote something down in my chart and told me to get dressed and that he would be back.

When Dr. Kastle returned to the room, he said, “Ms. Wilson, you do not have bromhidrosis, but I smell the odor of bromhidrosis coming from your vagina.”

“If I do not have bromhidrosis, how can you smell the odor coming from my vagina?” I asked.

“It’s a strong odor like bromhidrosis,” he said.

I told him I should have no odor and that I’d bathed that morning. “When I work, my coworkers comment about my body odor, and I always feel physically hot,” I explained to him that the odor emanated from my body as if I were running on a treadmill. “My vagina is sweaty, and I sweat under my arms, too,” I said.

He was writing in my folder as I spoke. “I want you to use Arm and Hammer deodorant,” he said. “I want you to use cornstarch in your vagina and under your arms.” He said I should take a fan to work with me, and when I sweat, I should go in the bathroom and lock the door, remove all my clothes, open my legs and arms wide, and let the fan cool me off. That made little sense to me. I told him I would not take a fan to work with me and get naked in the bathroom. He told me he was a doctor, and he did it, and sometimes you must do what you must do. I stood there looking at him in disbelief, thinking it was the dumbest advice I'd ever heard.

I left his office without thanking him. However, I purchased the Arm and Hammer deodorant and put it between my breasts and buttocks and under my arms. I also used cornstarch in my vagina. The odor was still there.

I made another appointment at the same dermatology clinic (Charity hospital Dermatology clinic) but asked to see a new dermatologist. I did not want to see Dr. Kastle again.

A month later, I got an appointment with Dr. Hoffman. I continued to work at the hotel, but I got a second job at a grocery store as a cashier. I asked my uncle to help me find a cheap one-bedroom apartment, and it took less than a week to find one for $180 a month. It was a shack, but I was getting closer to getting my daughter back. It was becoming clear that I might have to find the cure while my daughter lived with me. I did not know how long Ms. Tyler would keep Sherry, but I always thought I would get cured of my body odor first.

Luckily, my apartment had a bed, stove, and refrigerator. The property owner was a seventy-year-old woman, and all she asked was that I did not have company coming in and out of the apartment. I only had three friends: Lisa, Corey, and Linda. My sister was my best friend. I had to spend time around them for my own happiness. The more time I spent alone, the more I would fall into a deep depression.

I worked at the hotel and grocery store for the next three weeks. I moved into my apartment, and the first weekend after I moved in, Sherry and my nieces came over and spent the night. Sherry and I went shopping for shoes. I enjoyed my time with Sherry, but I was happy when it was time for her to return to Ms.

Tyler's house.

Five months after I started working at the grocery store, I had a mental breakdown. My life was not supposed to be like this. I was a housekeeper. I lived in a city I did not want to live in, and my daughter lived with a woman I did not know. I lost the energy to work two jobs. I had to get cured of this odor and go back to Chicago.

The night before my doctor's appointment, I wrote down everything I wanted the doctor to know. First, I needed to remove my sweat glands. Secondly, my body odor became fouler when my menstrual cycle came on every month. Thirdly, my body was experiencing hot flashes.

My body would become hot, and I would sweat heavily for no reason. And lastly, I would show him all the information I got from the books.

Corey came over later that night. When he came in, he asked me for a cup of water. I went into the kitchen to get him some water. I had left the information about bromhidrosis and the other papers on the bed. Corey came into the kitchen holding my documents.

"You think you smell foul?" he asked. It embarrassed me that he had read my papers, and I snatched them from his hands. He said, "Your ass is crazy."

I replied, "I am not a nasty person, and you know that, but my sweat glands are all messed up."

He came up behind me and hugged me tightly. As I put the papers under my bed, he whispered, "You think if you smelled bad, I would have sex with you?" Then he said, "You're right, your ass smells musty as hell."

I asked, "Do you smell me?"

He replied, "Hell no, girl. You do not smell."

At my doctor's appointment the next morning, I was anxious

to see Dr. Hoffman. I always thought, or at least hoped, that every new doctor would be the doctor to help me cure my odor.

Dr. Hoffman called me into the examination room. He already had my folder and said, "Ms. Wilson, I see you have been here before."

"Yes, I have," I said.

"Well, Ms. Wilson, I am standing right before you, and I do not smell you," he said.

I started crying. He gave me tissues and said, "Ms. Wilson, I will be right back." He returned five minutes later with four other student doctors and asked me questions.

"Do you smell the odor now?

"How many times a day do you smell the odor?"

One student asked me what kind of soap I used. As I answered the questions, some papers slipped from my hands and fell to the floor.

Dr. Hoffman said, "Oh, your important papers. Let me get them. We wouldn't want anything to happen to them now, would we?" This made him seem like a condescending asshole!

I asked him if I could see another dermatologist.

"Sure, but we all think you smell like a bed of roses," he said. I did not know what a bed of roses smelled like, but if they smelled like me, they would have smelled like shit.

Dr. Hoffman told me, "If you want to see another dermatologist, you can, but I am sure he or she will tell you the same thing: you do not smell."

I made an appointment. Thank God it was only two weeks later.

I made it to my appointment on time. This time, the lucky doctor was Dr. Blackman.

When Dr. Blackman walked into the exam room, I said, "Hello, Dr. Blackman, I would like you to look at the information

I have on a rare disorder that I think I may have. I relate to the condition of bromhidrosis. I do not know if you can smell me right now, but I found a book that may explain why some people smell me and others do not." I informed him that the book's authors were dermatologists, and that sweat gland removal surgery was the number one treatment for this condition.

"I would like to get my sweat glands removed," I said. Dr. Blackman asked me, "So where is this book?"

I looked at my chart in his hand as he scribbled something down; Dr. Blackman mentioned that I had seen Dr. Hoffman two weeks before. I wondered if Dr. Blackman felt the same way because his colleagues said they did not smell my odor. Deep inside, I wanted to cry. I asked him if he smelled me. He said he did not smell an odor. He asked me the name of the book.

I said, "*The Human Body Odor*."

Then he said, "You get the book and bring it to me, and I will read it." "You are a doctor; you can get the book before I can," I said.

"No, you can get the book," he told me.

I had to remain calm, but I was mad at Dr. Blackman.

I went by my sister's house to use her telephone; I could not afford to get a phone at my apartment. I called five libraries, all with no luck. Finally, at the sixth library, I called and asked the librarian how I could get a book that no library in New Orleans had. She asked me if I knew the author's name and when and where the book was published. I said I did. She told me to call the publishing company and tell them I would like to buy a copy of the book. I called the publishing company and asked the guy who answered the phone if they had a copy of the book *The Human Body Odor*.

"We stopped publishing the book. I could give you the names of some libraries with the book," he told me. He gave me the names and telephone numbers of four libraries in three different states. One of the libraries was in Chicago, where I had tried to steal the book from a few years before.

I called the first two libraries, but they did not have the book. The librarians said the book was out at this time. At the third library I called, the librarian inquired about the location of the previous library, where I knew the book was in stock. I told her it was a library in Chicago.

She said, "All you need to do is go to your local library with your library card and tell them you would like to borrow a book from a library in Chicago." She said it was a book-borrowing program that libraries had. I left for the library immediately. When I got to my local library, I applied for a library card, which I got right on the spot. I told the librarian I would like to borrow a book from Chicago. I handed her a piece of paper with the title of the book and the authors' names.

She looked at the paper and said, "You did all the computer work for me. All I need now is their telephone number." She punched some keys on the computer. The librarian called the University of Chicago Health and Science Library on Polk Street. As she talked, I stood on the other side of the counter, my heart racing. I knew the library in Chicago did not know my name, but I was nervous. The librarian hung up the phone after several minutes and looked at me.

"You are in luck. The book was damaged, but it is back in stock. It will be about two weeks before we get the book."

I gave her my sister's number and my work number. I called Dr. Blackman and informed him I would have the book in two weeks.

He said, "Good. When you get the book, bring it in and leave it with one of the nurses at the front desk and tell her the book is for me."

I said okay, but I was not putting that book in anybody's hand but Dr. Blackman's. My daughter and I continued to talk every week. I hoped the book would help Dr.

Blackman and me. A few times during those two weeks, while I waited for the book, I would wake up and feel nauseated, but I did not worry about it.

I called the library on the fourteenth business day. When I told the librarian my name, she said, "Ms. Wilson, I called you yesterday at the numbers you gave me. The book is here."

I immediately hung up the phone, ran to the bus stop, and went to the library. When I got to the library, I told the librarian I was so sorry for hanging up on her.

She said, "It's okay." She handed me the book and explained all the library's policies on book returns. I knew I was going to keep the book until I was cured.

The first thing I noticed about the book was that the color of the cover was different. The paragraph was not on the back of the book anymore, and the title was on the side of the book. I left the library and called Dr. Blackman from the first payphone I saw. I told him, "I have the book." I asked him if I could bring it to him that day.

He said, "You must hurry. The clinic is closing in thirty minutes." I was so worried I would miss him. I needed to get this book to him.

While on the bus, I took a pen and paper and wrote down certain pages and chapters I wanted Dr. Blackman to read. I wanted to take the book home and read it; it held the answers to getting my life back.

I got to the clinic; Dr. Blackman was still there. He received the book and papers. I pleaded with him to read the pages I wrote down.

He said, "I will call you on Monday. Before you go, I want to perform an excisional biopsy of a small, extracted slice of tissue from your armpit." He led me to an examination room and said he would return. He came back with another doctor. "Ms.

Wilson, this is Dr. Yates, and she will assist me with this extraction," he said. They numbed my left armpit, cut out a little piece of my tissue, and put it in a jar with a watery solution. Dr. Blackman told me he would call me on Monday.

It was Friday, and I had to work over the weekend. I was happy to have something to do.

It made the weekend go by faster.

On Monday, I went to the clinic at closing time and told the nurse I needed to see Dr. Blackman. She called him. I approached Dr. Blackman and said, "Hi, did you read the pages I told you to?"

"Yes, I read the book."

"Now, do you understand what I have been trying to tell you?" I asked. "You want your sweat glands removed?" he asked.

"Yes," I replied.

"You have to see a surgeon," he told me. He told me to make an appointment with the charity surgery clinic.

"You need to do it," I pleaded. "They will give me an appointment for two months from now."

"Just tell them you need to see a surgeon," he said.

"You need to give me my medical records to take over there; they will ask why I need the surgery," I said.

"Your medical records will go over there when you make the appointment," he assured me.

"What about the test results from the tissue extraction?" I asked.

He said I had an infection under my arm. "Is it bromhidrosis?" I asked. "Talk to the surgeon," he replied.

I was in luck. I got an appointment on the same day I called to make the appointment.

When I got to the surgery appointment, I signed in and noted sweat gland removal surgery as the reason for the visit. The nurse called me after twenty minutes. She asked me for my referral.

"My doctor said I did not need a referral, and my medical records would come here. He said I just needed to tell the surgeon that I wanted to get my sweat glands removed."

"That's not how it works," she replied. She told me to have a seat. After twenty minutes, the nurse and a doctor came to the front desk.

"Ms. Wilson, we do not have a folder on you. Why did your doctor tell you to come over here?"

I told her it was because I had a medical condition called bromhidrosis. "My doctor ran tests on me, and they showed the infection," I said.

"I have never heard of that condition," the doctor said. "I want to get my sweat glands removed," I explained.

"I still do not understand why he sent you here. We do not do that kind of surgery here. I am sorry, but you need to talk to your doctor and tell him we cannot help you," the doctor replied.

It was early, so I went to the dermatology clinic across the street. When I got to the clinic, I saw Dr. Blackman standing at the back, talking to another doctor. I was supposed to go to the front desk and check in with the nurse, but he was standing right there, so I just walked to the back of the clinic to speak with him.

"Excuse me, Dr. Blackman. The surgery clinic said they could not help me," I said.

Before he could say anything, a nurse from the front desk came charging toward me and said, "Carry, is everything okay? Come with me. You need to sign in to see Dr. Blackman." The nurse spoke to me as if I was out of control.

But Dr. Blackman said, "It is okay. I will see her," motioning for me to enter an examination room. I rolled my eyes at the nurse as I walked toward the room. Dr. Blackman asked me if I wanted to get my sweat glands removed.

"Yes, I want to stop this odor." I handed him the

bromhidrosis medication list and asked him, "If you prescribed me any of these medications, would they kill me?" He looked at the list.

"Of course not," he said, frowning.

"Well, why can't you just give them to me to see if they will stop the body odor?" I asked. I told him I specifically wanted to take anticholinergic drugs, but he told me immediately that he does not write prescriptions for anticholinergic drugs for anyone. He would write me a prescription for a topical solution. I agreed and asked if anticholinergic drugs were the only oral treatment for bromhidrosis. He said yes and wrote me the prescription for the topical solution. I went to the drugstore and got the solution immediately.

I went home and shaved all the hair off my vaginal wall and under my armpits. The topical solution had a strong acid scent. I applied it to my vaginal wall and armpits; the solution burned my skin, but I continued using it.

I got the book back from Dr. Blackman and started reading it. The book confirmed a lot of things I already knew. The book stated that the odor of bromhidrosis became worse when a woman's menstrual cycle came on, just like I had told the doctors. My menstrual cycle smelled like a dead rat. The odor did not come from inside my vagina but from my vaginal wall, and my urine smelled bad too.

I continued using the topical solutions for a week. At first, the solution worked. It would suppress the odor for several hours, but the odor always came back. After a week of using the topical solution, it burned and irritated my skin.

On Monday, I returned to the clinic and told the nurse I needed to see Dr. Blackman. She asked if I had an appointment.

I said, "No."

She told me to have a seat as she rolled her eyes at me. It was the same nurse from that day in the hallway.

Dr. Blackman called me after twenty minutes, and when we got into the examination room, he asked me if I still had the odor. I told him I still had it and showed him how the topical solution made blisters under my arm and irritated my vaginal wall. He told me I was not supposed to put the solution near my vagina. "I will give you a different topical solution," he said.

"Could you please just do the surgery?" I asked.

"Make an appointment for next Monday, and I will remove a little sweat gland from under both of your arms to see if it relieves the odor."

I was so happy that I cried. My nightmare was finally over. I was getting the number one treatment for bromhidrosis. I made the appointment, but two days later, I realized that my menstrual cycle had not come on for the month, and it was the time of the month when my cycle should be stopping. This was unusual, as I was never late. I never even missed my cycle. I started thinking about the worst. Corey and I did not have sex a lot. We always used condoms, but there were a couple of occasions when the condoms broke. I did not want him to impregnate me.

I walked to the drugstore and bought a pregnancy test with two tests. The result was positive. After nine years, I was pregnant with my second child. This was the wrong time, and I felt so bad because I knew I should not be pregnant.

I caught the bus to Lisa's house the following afternoon. I told her I was pregnant and did not know what to do. She asked if I had told anyone else that I was pregnant. I told her I had not told Corey, my sister, or Sherry yet. I needed time to figure things out. If I told my sister, I knew she would tell me it was stupid to let myself get pregnant, as I had always told her I wanted to be cured and get my life and Sherry back.

"I am going to call Corey later today, and my sister is going to be mad at me," I said.

The second pregnancy test was in my purse, so I took the test to make sure I was pregnant. The second test was positive, too.

"Well, I am pregnant," I said to Lisa.

I finally paged Corey and put "911" behind the number so he would know I was paging him for an emergency.

Lisa asked if I wanted her to stay in the room while I talked to Corey. "I am nervous, but I can do this," I told her.

The phone rang, and Corey picked it up. I said hello, and before Corey could say anything, I said, "I am pregnant!"

He asked, "Are you serious?"

I said yes. "But you have so many things wrong with you; will the baby have medical problems?" he replied. I did not know what to say because I agreed with him; I did not want to be pregnant with everything happening in my life and my body. What if I passed this odor on to my unborn child? I was terrified, so I apologized to Corey and told him I would talk to him the next day.

(Present day 2025: Neither of my children has TMAU/body odor.) The next day, I visited my sister. I knocked on her door and walked into her apartment. As my sister came to answer the door, she looked at me and said, "What is wrong? I can see it in your face. Something is wrong. Another doctor said they did not smell you?" she asked.

"I am pregnant," I told her.

My sister just stood there in disbelief. "Girl, stop playing," she said. "I am pregnant," I repeated.

"You wait all these years, with all the other shit you must deal with, and you decide to get pregnant now?" she asked.

"I did not try to get pregnant on purpose. Corey and I always had safe sex," I explained. She shook her head. "Not too safe." She asked if I had told Sherry.

"No, and I will not tell her right now."

"You are going to have the baby?" she asked.

I do not know what to do. It surprised me that my sister was more concerned about how I felt and wasn't mad that I was pregnant.

I called Dr. Blackman the next morning and informed him that I was pregnant.

He said, "I cannot do the sweat gland removal surgery while you are pregnant." I asked him if he could prescribe another type of topical solution for me. He said he would phone in the prescription and I should contact him after I had given birth to discuss whether having the surgery was necessary. *Of course, it would still be necessary after I give birth*, I thought to myself.

I got the topical solution, and again, it worked, but then I started getting blisters under my arms. Dr. Blackman told me not to use the solution on my vagina, but I used it on my vaginal wall. The solution irritated my vagina again, so I had to stop worrying about the odor and relax until after I had my baby; then, I could move forward with the surgery.

I left my sister's house later that afternoon, and Corey came to my apartment that night to try to convince me to have an abortion. He told me he was worried that the baby would be sick, and he was not ready for the baby. I had to tell Corey with conviction that I did not want to talk about having an abortion. I was having a baby. Corey was upset but realized it was my body and my choice. I had sex with Corey that night before he left my apartment. As much as his words hurt me, I loved him and did not want to go through this alone. Abortion was never an option. I did not have the baby because it was the right or wrong thing to do; the baby, my baby, would not judge me no matter what I smelled like. I also thought whatever was causing the odor would stop me from getting pregnant. (I was wrong)

The next day, I went over to my sister's house to call Sherry after she got home from school, and the first thing she asked was, "Mama, are you pregnant?"

I asked her, "Who told you that?"

“Ms. Tyler told me, ‘Your mother is giving you a little brother or sister.’” I became enraged. I knew Lisa had told Ms. Tyler I was pregnant, and it got back to Sherry.

I told Sherry, “Yes, I am pregnant.”

She begged, “Mama, I want to come back home.” I replied, “I am going to call you right back.”

I called Lisa and said a lot of unpleasant curse words. I told her I did not appreciate her telling anyone about my business, and I told her we were no longer friends. I liked Lisa; she had been genuinely nice to me and my daughter. She did more for me than some of my family members. I appreciated her, but I had to move on. I have not spoken to Lisa since 1999. During my pregnancy, I stopped working because of morning sickness. For the next eight months, life seemed a little more normal.

Sherry came to live with me, and we moved in with my sister. I tried to read and understand the book, *The Human Body Odor*. However, I skipped some chapters that I did not understand. I continued to visit libraries and read other books on bromhidrosis. While at the library, I sometimes came across other conditions with body odor as a symptom, but I related to bromhidrosis more.

Corey visited me off and on during those eight months to see how my pregnancy was going.

I gave birth to my son, Corey Jr., in 2000 by C-section. After I gave birth, my menstrual cycle started immediately. My hospital room smelled like hot garbage. I opened the window in my room as wide as I could.

When the nurse came in to let me feed my baby, she said, “Ms. Wilson, close this window; it’s too cool in here for the baby.”

Corey Sr. and one of his female friends came to see his son, and his friend mentioned that my room smelled horrible. I remember thinking I could not escape this odor, even on a joyous day.

When baby Corey Jr. and I came home from the hospital, my daughter was so happy to see her new little brother, but my sister said, "Carry, we need to have a serious conversation." She told me she and her boyfriend were getting back together, and she was moving out. She said I could stay in the apartment but had to get a job to pay the rent and bills. "I am not moving right now, but in a week or two. I will pay the rent for the month, but just like Daddy told you, let this odor go and get a job; you have two kids to take care of now," she continued.

"Thank you," I said. "I will get a job, but I can never give up on my fight to eliminate this odor."

THE FIGHT

In June of 2000, I went to the dermatology clinic and asked to speak to Dr. Blackman. When he was available, we stood in the waiting room talking. I informed him that I had given birth to my son and that I was ready for surgery.

Dr. Blackman asked if my son's father had ever complained about my body odor. "He has said he never smelled me, but I think he can," I replied.

"You can return on Monday, and I will perform the surgery," Dr. Blackman said.

When I returned to the clinic the following Monday, I told the nurse I was there to see Dr.

Blackman.

"Dr. Blackman is not coming into the clinic today. Are you sure the appointment was for today?" she asked.

"Yes. Dr. Blackman is supposed to be performing surgery on me today," I told her. "I do not have you in my appointment book," she replied.

"He told me last week to just come on Monday," I said.

She told me to take a seat and that a doctor would call me shortly. I sat down. I did not overreact, but I was concerned that Dr. Blackman was not at the clinic.

Eventually, Dr. Yates came out and called me. I recognized her as the doctor who had extracted my tissue with Dr. Blackman. She led me into the examination room. I looked around the room and did not see my chart or any surgical supplies.

"Hi, Ms. Wilson," she said. "Do you remember me?"

"Yes," I told her. "Dr. Blackman is supposed to take my sweat glands out today."

"Ms. Wilson," she said. "Dr. Blackman will not take your sweat glands out, nor will any other doctor in this clinic." Her tone was aggressive; it ripped right through me. It was powerful; she made me feel like a small child as she told me to get myself a bar of Dial soap and a bottle of perfume and get on with my life. I just sat there in disbelief. I was having flashbacks to when Dr. Walsh threatened to take me to court and get a judgment that would give him the right to prescribe me psychological medication.

"I do not use scented soap or perfume," I said. "The scents of some products do not mix well with my body odor."

"Ms. Wilson, I'm so sorry you are so upset, but you must get on with your life," she said. I told her I would write a letter to the NAACP (National Association for the

Advancement of Colored People), and she told me to do whatever I wanted.

I left the clinic in shambles. Why had Dr. Blackman said he would perform the surgery and then changed his mind without telling me?

I wrote letters to the NAACP, Oprah Winfrey, and her best friend, Gayle, *Essence Magazine*, 20/20, news stations, women's organizations, and the American Association of Dermatology, all with no response. However, the Dermatology Association and the NAACP wrote back to me, but they were no help, so I wrote them a second letter.

Shortly after the visit to Dr. Blackman's office, I became suicidal and was admitted into the Charity Hospital's mental ward. I always felt better once I was away from society and had been admitted into the ward. I was there for four nights and five days.

When I got out of the mental ward, my fight with the doctors resumed, but I had a new game plan. First, I asked my auntie if Sherry could come and live with her for a couple of months. She said yes. Then Corey Jr. went to stay with his father.

Second, I asked my sister Candice and her friend Linda to write an honest letter to the doctor, expressing what I smelled like. I asked them to sign the letters and include their phone numbers.

Third, I planned to interact differently with doctors from then on. From 1996-1999, I let my body odor take over my emotions and my life. I cried often. I was not getting through to doctors; I was weak. In mid-2000, I vowed to be stronger. I needed to dress classier and speak like I had been to college.

I sat there thinking, *why am I not reaching these doctors? What am I doing wrong?*

That's when it hit me; I had to stop telling new doctors that the doctors I had seen said they did not smell an odor coming from me. I had to stop breaking down and crying in front of doctors; they knew I was an emotional wreck. I had to get another job—or be homeless.

I got a job as a housekeeper at another hotel. I lasted three months there before my coworkers ran me off the job. After that, I got a job as a security guard. At that job, I could work alone—any job with minimal contact with coworkers was better. I worked as a security guard for several months. In total, I worked at and quit six or more jobs throughout 2000.

In 2001, I continued writing letters to health officials. I begged the American Association of Dermatology to intervene in the neglectful healthcare I had received from dermatologists in New Orleans. In the letters, I stressed that I had been repeatedly misdiagnosed with chemical imbalances that I did not have. Dermatologists had repeatedly stated that I did not have a body odor, but I had a medical condition that caused me to have a foul body. The American Association of Dermatology wrote back and informed me that they did not have dermatologists who worked at the association; however, they had a membership of over ten thousand dermatologists. (I could only wait and hope for a response from the other associations I wrote to.)

In 2001, I saw a patient advocate at a charity hospital and I asked for help in getting the doctors to help me, but there was still no help. I saw two more dermatologists before the end of the year and asked them both if they could prescribe anticholinergic drugs for me; one of them said he did not write prescriptions for that medicine, and the other doctor said he would not prescribe anticholinergic drugs because there was no reason for me to take them.

In 2002, my children and I were evicted from our apartment as I was broke and unemployed again because of my body odor. During the years when my body odor had been undiagnosed, my children and I stayed in homeless shelters, which was a horrible experience. Most women in the shelters made direct, vicious comments to my face about my body odor, and I would leave in a day or two.

I picked myself up again and completed a six-week course to become a certified nursing assistant (CNA). It wasn't easy to make it through those classes. I had to sit inside a small classroom with twenty other women for two hours, five days a week, but I made it through the comments and the laughing behind my back about my body odor.

I did not realize how much physical labor went into working in healthcare. I would sweat profusely while at work. Getting my certification helped me stay employed longer. Still, once the comments from my coworkers became too vicious, I would continue to quit nursing jobs and get others at another nursing home.

In 2002, I was admitted into the charity hospital mental ward for the second time because I was exhausted, depressed, and suicidal. I was ready to give up. I could not take comments at work anymore; they hurt too much. I was tired of filling out job applications. Being depressed made me physically sick. I had gained over eighty pounds, and my hair was damaged beyond repair. I often sat around looking as if I were in a daze. I also started feeling like my surroundings were unreal, like I was in a dream world. I questioned my sanity. I thought maybe the doctors were right; the odor was in my head. Still, I knew they were wrong.

I lied to the psychiatrist; I told him I was ready to accept that I had a mental illness that made me delusional about having an odor coming from my body. I was prepared to take medication and see a psychiatrist regularly. I needed financial help because I could not keep a roof over my kids' heads. The lights in my apartment got turned off every month, and I told the psychiatrist I thought my daughter hated me and wished she had a normal mother, one who did not smell bad.

My daughter was ashamed of how I looked and smelled and she hated that she and her brother did not have adequate clothing, but I tried my best to buy them things between jobs.

Sometimes, I could quit a job and get another within a week, but sometimes, two months would go by and I would remain without a job.

The psychiatrist told me I needed to go to the Social Security office and apply for a mental disability check. He also gave me a referral to a clinic for mentally ill patients. I hated to lie to anyone about my body odor, but the doctors gave me no choice: I had to lie to get the check every month. I would use some of the money from the check to pay for bus fare, continue my fight with doctors, and go to the library to do research. I never told the psychiatrists I was still searching for a cure for my body odor.

By late 2002, I had worked several more jobs while waiting for a decision from the Social Security Administration about my disability claim. My children and I moved back and forth between my mother and sister.

Finally, the American Association of Dermatology responded to my letters. I requested assistance from the association with finding a dermatologist who had treated someone with bromhidrosis, and they mailed me a referral to Dr. Swartz of the Charity Dermatology Clinic. I called the clinic and asked to speak with Dr. Swartz.

"My name is Carry Wilson," I explained. "I wrote a letter to the American Association of Dermatology, asking them to help me find a dermatologist who had treated a patient for bromhidrosis. They sent me a letter with your name and number."

Dr. Swartz told me to come the next morning at 9:00 a.m. and to bring the letter. I was usually eager to see a new doctor, but I was worried that he worked at the charity dermatology clinic where Dr. Blackman worked, and I knew he would not help me.

Physically, my body has given up. I was tired, but mentally, I still had hope to keep fighting, so I thought, *"Here I go again."*

I made it to the clinic and asked to see Dr. Swartz. The nurse told me to sign in and take a seat. A few minutes later, a doctor called me to the front desk.

"Hi, Ms. Wilson. I am Dr. Swartz. Do you have the letter?" I gave him the letter; he read it and told me to take a seat. After thirty minutes, Dr. Blackman called me, and as I walked toward him, I wondered why he had called me. I did not want to see him again. He pointed to the exam room. Four other doctors were in the room when we entered.

Sitting and looking at all the other doctors, I asked Dr. Blackman, "Where is Dr.

Swartz?"

"He said he will join us soon," I was told.

I asked Dr. Blackman if he could put me in a room without air conditioning; I told him it would help them smell my odor if I got hot and sweaty. I also told him I would like to try anticholinergic drugs to see if they would stop my body odor.

"Let's wait for Dr. Swartz to come," he said.

When Dr. Swartz came into the room, Dr. Blackman said, "Ms. Wilson would like to be put in a room without air conditioning. She thinks it will help us smell her body odor."

Dr. Swartz replied, "That won't be necessary."

Dr. Blackman continued, "She would also like to try some anticholinergic drugs."

Dr. Swartz asked me why I wanted to take anticholinergic drugs. I told him, as I had told the other doctors, that in the book *The Human Body Odor*, dermatologists treated patients from whom they did not smell an odor; however, they had other tests done, and anticholinergics were successful in treating these patients for bromhidrosis.

Dr. Swartz said okay. He wrote me a prescription for twenty pills; I was supposed to take two pills a day. He said he would see me in two weeks.

I shaved all the hair off my body, took pills daily, and caked corn starch and deodorant into my armpits and vagina twice a day.

Like the topical solution, the anticholinergic pills initially stopped my body odor, but the odor always returned. I was so depressed. I saw two more doctors who prescribed anticholinergic drugs for me because I showed them the empty prescription bottle Dr. Swartz had prescribed for me. One of them was Dr. Roberts, a doctor I had seen before who refused to prescribe anticholinergic drugs for me because he said, "I did not have a body odor." Still, he gave me a prescription once I gave him the bottle.

When I told Dr. Roberts, I would make an appointment to

come back and see him in two weeks, he said, "No, you do not need to see me again."

I felt like no doctor wanted to be bothered by me. They all felt the anticholinergic drugs were not stopping the odor because there was no odor to stop, but the thought of having this body odor for the rest of my life made me sick. Not getting diagnosed made me mad. I knew I had to get my sweat glands removed.

In late 2002, I lived with my sister until I received my disability checks, and with my first check, I got my apartment. It was a one-bedroom piece of shit, but it was somewhere for me and my kids to live. Getting the check every month took two percent of my depression away because it eliminated the homelessness that had followed my children and me around like a bad odor (pun intended!)

I paid my rent and light bill monthly for the next few months and got food stamps to keep food in the refrigerator. Doing these things gave me a little strength to fight the doctors.

My sister had a friend named Terry who had gone to college. She was intelligent and business minded. I asked her if she could go on the computer and try to find a surgeon who performed sweat gland removal surgery for people with bromhidrosis. I gave her all the paperwork I had on the condition. She took one day to provide me with the name and telephone number of a doctor who performed the surgery not just for bromhidrosis but also for a condition called hyperhidrosis. Hyperhidrosis is when a person sweats profusely but has no body odor.

However, the authors of *The Human Body Odor* hypothesized that hyperhidrosis is almost always accompanied by bromhidrosis. My sweat smelled bad, and I sweated profusely most days.

I called the surgeon in Chicago, who told me to send him a copy of my medical records, and he would tell me if he could perform the surgery. What I did next was illegal and stupid, but I was desperate—I altered a few of my medical records. I used white-out on my records anywhere the doctor wrote, "No odor noticed," the word "phobia," etc. I made a copy of my medical records so that all the surgeons could see that I had been seeing doctors who said I had bromhidrosis. My altered medical and original documents are at the end of this book.

I mailed my (altered) records to the doctor, who mailed me a welcome packet. He told me he could perform the surgery for just under $3,000.

I did not have the money and decided I had to work to get it, but I was mentally terrified about going back to work. The people would talk badly about me. (Verbal Violence) I was strong, but I could not take being around people. I had developed a phobia of being around people other than my sister, her kids, or my kids.

The surgeon said my insurance would not pay for the surgery unless my doctor said I needed it for medical purposes. I had to find a dermatologist whom I had not seen before who accepted my insurance. At this point, I have seen over 25 doctors.

I was lucky. I found a new dermatologist, Dr. Wagdon. When I saw him, I told him I had bromhidrosis, and I showed him all the paperwork I had on bromhidrosis and my altered medical records. I impressed him with my research. I told him I wanted to get my sweat glands surgically removed and needed a referral from a doctor in New Orleans. He looked shocked and said he did not think the surgery was a good idea.

He said, "Let me tell you why," as he demonstrated how some people who have had the surgery end up with deformed armpits because a nerve was cut during the surgery.

I said, "I don't care. I will take my chances."

He warned me, "Ms. Wilson, please ensure you have done all your research. Make sure you have left no stone unturned before you have the surgery."

I told him, "I have been trying to get cured since 1996."

He asked, "Before you get the surgery, will you try an anticholinergic drug?"

I told him I had tried them, but they did not work. He asked me if I had tried a certain kind, and the name did not sound familiar, so I said, "Okay, I will try the pills." I tried the pills but did not want to, and they did not stop the odor like I knew they wouldn't.

I returned to Dr. Wagdon's office two weeks later and this time, I saw Dr. Sherman. Dr. Sherman asked, "Ms. Wilson, did the pills stop the odor?"

I said no.

He said, "Dr. Wadgon and I want to know if you would try Botox injections. You say the odor is coming from your armpits. The injection will stop you from sweating in your armpits." He explained the whole sweat and odor process. I hoped the injections would stop the odor.

I asked him, "What about my vaginal wall?"

He replied, "Ms. Wilson, we cannot give you Botox injections anywhere in your vaginal area."

I said I had to ask.

The injections stopped me from sweating in my armpits but did not stop the odor.

After the injections didn't work, I knew Dr. Sherman did not want to give me a referral for surgery. I fell into a deep depression; I did not want to return to work to get the money for the surgery. Every day, I woke up to the same scene. The walls and curtains in my apartment smelled like me, like shit and mildew. I hated waking up. I was thankful my daughter spent most of her time at my auntie's house, and I let my son stay the night at his grandparents' house for as many nights as they would let him. I did not go out; I had no life. I was numb. I was in a dark place, and I started feeling like I had in Chicago when I was feeling suicidal. I did not want to cook, smile, or be a mother.

One day, my sister came by my apartment and said, "Carry, I have an idea. This is what we can do. You and I can get an apartment. All you have to do is give me all your food stamps every month. You take $300 from your disability check every month until you save the money for the surgery. You must buy things for yourself and the kids, so save $300 a month."

"What made you do this?" I asked.

"Carry, you look like you've had a hard life. It's all in your face. I want my sister back. If I had the money, I would give it to you, but save it and get your surgery," she cried.

In 2003, my children and I moved into an apartment with my sister and her kids so I could save up the money for my sweat gland removal surgery. Everything went according to plan for a few months, but I was severely depressed and needed a fix, so I went to the library. Going to the library to read old or current information on bromhidrosis was like medication for me mentally; it reassured me I was not crazy and that I would get cured one day.

I went to the library and asked the librarian if she could pull up the bromhidrosis website.

There was a lot of current information on the site. As I read and navigated from page to page, I came across a statement that read, "Other problems and conditions to be considered: Trimethylaminuria, Fish Odor Syndrome." When I read that statement, I thought nothing of it.

I took notes from the website. I punched many keys on the computer but did not know what I was doing. For the time being, I gave up. I had copied enough valuable information for the day.

As I left the library, the librarian said, "Miss, do not forget your printouts." She saw that I was confused so she said, "Your printouts on the computer, the information you were just reading." I walked up to the front desk and looked at the papers. I told her I had not tried to print out the information, but I was lucky; it was the first of the month, and I had the money to buy the copies.

I got home, gathered all my information on bromhidrosis, and read all the papers I had. I would do this at least three times a year to make sure I had not missed anything that could help me. It would usually take me a couple of days to read all the information I had collected over the years. At this point, I was reading everything I'd collected from June 1996 to March 2003.

As I read my papers, if I came across other conditions with body odor as a symptom, I would read up on them. If I related to one of them, I would ask a doctor to test me for it.

I successfully convinced doctors to test me for diabetes, thyroid problems, hormone imbalances, and amino acid levels. Some of these conditions were possibilities for the source of my body odor. All my tests came back negative.

I sat on my bed, reading the information I had gotten from the library. Other problems and conditions to be considered included fish Odor Syndrome (Trimethylaminuria). Again, I did not react to this statement.

A few months later, I read all the information again. I had no life. All I did was watch TV, cry, and read, but when I read that statement that time, a light bulb went off in my head. *I should go to the library for more information on this condition,* I thought.

I asked the librarian to pull up information on the condition of trimethylaminuria, but there was not a lot of useful information on the computer. I asked the librarian if she had any research advice on rare disorders, and she told me to contact an organization called The National Organization for Rare Disorders (NORD). I got the organization's phone number, called them, and asked them to send me more information on trimethylaminuria. It took about a week for me to get the only information NORD had on TAMU in 2003.

As I read the symptoms, I started crying. For the first time in years, I was reading about a condition I could have; something other than bromhidrosis. I read the information on this condition about how eating certain foods can make a person physically hot; this explained the hot flashes I had been experiencing for years. People with this condition smell like fish, feces, urine, and other foul odors. That would explain why I smelled like so many foul odors. I had to calm down; just because I related to the condition did not mean I had it.

There was a contact number for Dr. Pratt, who evaluated patients for this condition. I called him. I said, "Hi, Dr. Pratt. My name is Carry Wilson, and I may have trimethylaminuria." I could not pronounce the condition correctly, so Dr. Pratt encouraged me to say TMAU.

"Fish odor syndrome is the old name for the condition. Trimethylaminuria is the new name, and TMAU is an abbreviation," he told me.

"I would like to be tested for TMAU," I said. He asked me why I thought I had TMAU.

"For the last seven years, I have smelled like urine, rotten fish, and other foul odors," I replied. "I have seen many doctors who gave me good hygiene advice, but the odor did not go away." Of course, doctors had not given me good hygiene advice, but I would not tell Dr. Pratt that. I also would not tell him that the doctors I had seen said they did not smell an odor from me. I was already obsessed with taking this test, and nothing would stop me.

Dr. Pratt got straight to the point. He told me to write him a letter telling him why I wanted to take the test, and he said, "Put it in the letter that you talked to me today."

I asked, "How much does a test like this cost?" He said, "$250."

I was happy! He gave me the mailing address, and I said

thank you. I wrote and mailed the letter on the same day I spoke to him. He said I should hear from him within in two weeks.

While I waited to hear from Dr. Pratt, I called NORD. I asked them if they could send me more information on TMAU, but I was told by the operator that they had already sent me all the material they had. She suggested I go to my local library, and I did.

I discovered there was no cure for TMAU, but chemists and scientists were working on a cure as well as treatment options at the Monell Chemical Senses Center.

I learned that TMAU was not contagious and that I would not die from having the condition if I had it. The good news was that there were treatment options for this condition.

The more I read, the more I tried to convince myself that I had this condition.

Two weeks after I wrote the letter to Dr. Pratt, I was at home when someone knocked on the apartment's front door.

My niece said, "Auntie Carry, someone is at the door for you." It was the UPS man. I asked, "Who are you looking for?"

He replied, "Carry Wilson," handing me a big box and a paper form to sign. I asked him, "What is this?"

"Did you order something?" he asked.

I said no. I took the box, ran to my room, and found a letter attached to it. It was from Dr.

Pratt; it was a kit for me to test myself for TMAU. I called Dr. Pratt as the letter instructed.

He said, "Ms. Wilson, follow the directions for taking the test, and the day you send the test back to me completed by overnight mail, call me."

The test consisted of mixing and drinking an ingredient called choline into some milk or orange juice. If I had trimethylaminuria, the choline would produce an odor in my body. When I took the test, I had to drink the choline and urinate in four little cups for four days and four nights and then put those containers in the freezer to freeze overnight. I had to buy a Styrofoam container and dry ice. Once all four containers were full, I had to put them in the Styrofoam container with the dry ice and ship them back to Dr. Pratt overnight.

I waited two weeks to take the test until my menstrual cycle came on. I knew my body odor was always strongest during that time of the month. The wait gave me time to practice taking the test.

Finally, my cycle came on, and I took the test. Once I completed the test, I sent it off overnight with a money order for $250. I called Dr. Pratt the next day, and he said he had received my test kit and would contact me as soon as he got the results.

I waited three days and called Dr. Pratt to ask if he had received my results. He said, "Ms. Wilson, the test takes six to seven weeks to complete."

"Oh, my God. I thought it was like any other test, three days," I said.

"No. You can relax for a few weeks, and I will call you as soon as I get your results," he told me.

I was so disappointed that I had to wait so long.

My sister said, "You have been waiting for over seven years. A couple of weeks will not be that long of a wait. Carry, you must stop thinking you have this condition for sure. What if you don't have it? All I know is that if you do not have this condition, I am through with you and the whole odor thing." I have never asked my sister what exactly she meant when she said she would be through with me, and I never want to know.

Six weeks passed and finally, I got a release form in the mail from a clinic, instructing me to sign and mail the release back so the facility could release my test results to Dr. Pratt. I signed the release form, and before I sent it back, I noticed Beverly Frank's signature and telephone number at the top of the release form.

I decided to call Ms. Frank, and when she answered the phone. I said, "Hi, Ms. Frank.

My name is Carry Wilson, and I got a letter from your office."

"Well, yes, Ms. Wilson. Just sign the release form and send it back in the envelope we provided," she instructed.

I asked her if my test was complete. "No, there is someone in front of you. We should start your test on Monday," she replied.

It was Friday. I was happy. In two days, they would start my test.

Monday came and went. I called Ms. Frank the following Thursday. She informed me she would mail my test results the following Monday. She told me if I did not understand my results, I could call her, and she would go over them with me. I asked if she knew what my test results were right then.

She said, "I can't discuss your results until you get them."

The weekend went by fast. I went to bed early every night so the days could come quickly. Monday came and went. I let my daughter stay home from school on Thursday.

My daughter, Sherry, was twelve years old and knew I was waiting for the test results which would explain why I smelled so bad. My daughter and my sister wanted to know the results as much as I did. My daughter needed her mother back, and my sister wanted her sister back, too.

THE RESULTS

Finally, my test results should arrive today. Our mail carrier came every day between 10:30 a.m. and 11:00 a.m. I told my sister at 10:00 a.m., “I am going into my bedroom. Open the results and read them; if they are positive, bang on my door; and if they are negative, leave me alone.”

She went outside to wait for the mail to be delivered. At 10:40 a.m., I was sitting on my bed when my sister opened the door and shook her head. “No mail,” she said. I could not believe it.

My sister said, “Girl, it will be here tomorrow.” Friday came and went, and still no results. I called Ms. Frank back and asked if she had mailed back my results.

“I told you I was mailing them off on Monday, and I did. Have patience, Ms. Wilson,” she said.

By Saturday, I still had not gotten the results. On Monday, the kids did not have school.

I was sitting outside waiting for the mail carrier at 11:00 a.m. When he walked straight past my apartment, I asked, “No mail for me today?”

He replied, “Not today.”

I went into the apartment, sat on the couch, and started crying.

“Carry, sometimes it takes a little longer to get mail from other states,” my sister said.

I did not want to hear that. I wanted to know if I had this monster in my body. That was when it hit me; I remembered that Ms. Frank said when I got my test results back, she would go over them with me if I did not understand them.

I wrote my social security number and birthday on a piece of paper. I asked my sister to call Ms. Frank and say, "Hi, Ms. Frank, this is Carry Wilson, and I do not understand my test results." I was too nervous to make the call, so my sister made it for me.

It was a beautiful, warm day. My sister and I went outside with the cordless phone. My sister was leaning back on her car, facing me. I was six feet away from her, pacing back and forth as I heard my sister say, "Hi, Ms. Frank."

I was biting my nails; I felt like I would throw up from being so nervous. I watched my sister talk and nod her head. She did not look at me. I could tell nothing from her facial expression. I did not know what to think, and then my sister hung up the phone and nodded her head up and down.

"You got it. You have TMAU!" she exclaimed. I almost fell on my buttocks; I was blown away. My sister and I cried and jumped up and down. The kids ran out of the house.

My daughter asked, "You got it?"

"Yes, baby," I replied as I hugged and kissed her. I had it. I had a body odor. I was not crazy, and I had been right all the time.

My sister said, "Girl, call Ms. Frank back. When she said your test results were positive, I just hung up the phone."

I called her back immediately. "I am sorry, Ms. Frank, but my son pulled the cord out of the wall."

"Well, yes, like I was saying, you have TMAU, and your levels were very high," she said.

"I am not surprised; I smell bad," I said. I thanked her and called Dr. Pratt and told him I had tested positive. He said he knew because he had received my test results in the mail that morning. Dr. Pratt informed me he would send me some supplements called Derifil (also known as chlorophyllin). Derifil supplements are a treatment for TMAU. Dr. Pratt said he was sending me information on foods high in choline and steps I could take to control my body odor.

He also gave me the telephone number of a woman named Karen who lived in LA who ran a TMAU support group. Dr. Pratt thought it would be a good idea for me to contact Karen for guidance.

I thanked Dr. Pratt and told him it was as if God had led me to him. "No, Ms. Wilson. I am just doing my job," he said.

I asked Dr. Pratt if he had TMAU, and he said no.

I called Karen. "Hi, my name is Carry, and I just discovered I have TMAU. Dr. Pratt gave me your number."

She said, "You must be relieved to know you have TMAU."

I told her it had been a long fight. I told her the doctors would not go beyond the office and go on the computer to look up the information I gave them. Karen talked about the difficulties of getting diagnosed with TMAU. She even knew of a person who had spent well over $10,000 trying to discover why they smelled so bad. I shared with Karen that my result levels were high and that I did not understand TMAU.

I asked her, "What is this? What the hell is TMAU?" She used a lot of medical jargon, and I stopped her mid-sentence and said, "I am going to need you to repeat that in English."

She laughed and said, "Think of it this way. When you eat, your body does not break down certain foods properly, and because of that, your body produces a foul body odor."

"Wow, simply wow!" I exclaimed. I also asked Karen if I could get my body odor down to undetectable levels.

Getting the odor level down to undetectable levels is

possible. I still have the odor, but it is not loud, and I could sit next to someone, and the odor they smell coming off me is not offensive. I could take the funky, foul scent out of the odor by eliminating certain foods from my diet and taking supplements like Derifil, probiotics, and Riboflavin (vitamin B2). Derifil and other supplemental treatment results are debatable among body odor sufferers. I, personally, do not take Derifil because it made my odor worse.

"Yes," Karen replied. She told me she did not take Derifil because it was too expensive. She ate a healthy, low-choline diet, and she exercised every day. She said exercising had helped control the odor of TMAU.

After talking to Karen, I felt good; she gave me hope that I would get my body odor down to undetectable levels.

The day after I tested positive for TMAU, I walked outside, and, for the first time in seven years – a beautiful, sunny day – felt like a beautiful, sunny day. It was as if a cloud had been lifted from me emotionally. I felt different. I was finally optimistic about my future.

THE AFTERMATH

It was late 2003. It had been several months since I tested positive for trimethylaminuria.

It had been an up-and-down battle for me and my children. While I was the one who had the odor, my children continued to go through hell with me, especially my daughter. I learned that diet and exercise were pivotal in my fight against TMAU so I tried to change my eating habits, but my depression drove my food addiction.

At the gym, people would make faces and discuss my body odor, and I continued to be embarrassed.

I worked off and on, but I could not always afford Derifil. I would learn that certain ingredients in most of the foods on the planet, like soy, lecithin, soybeans, salt, etc., directly affected the foulness of my body odor.

I went on a binge and ate a lot of fruit and salads to bring my odor level down. Some people with foul body odor will notice when the foulness of their body odor decreases. I was doing a decent job dieting and exercising. Still, sometimes, I craved chicken, pizza, or junk food. (anything other than salad). I did not understand why, with everything I had been through, I would dare eat foods I knew would make me smell foul. I would go back and forth, eating foods that would bring my body odor and foulness up and down. I frequently prayed to God to help me stop bingeing on these foods.

There was so much going on. I tried to sue some doctors in court for failure to diagnose, medical negligence, and abusive and neglectful health care, but I could not get a lawyer to represent me. I wrote letters to the NAACP, the Rainbow Push Coalition, and Dr. Phil and his wife, Robin, asking them to help me fight against these doctors in court. I knew I had to fight power with power. The doctors were powerful; I was a poor Black woman from the ghetto.

I got no response from Dr. Phil or the NAACP, and Rainbow Push told me by phone that they could not help me in court because I had filed papers before I got a lawyer. I understood little of what was being said or mailed from the court, but I knew I had a court date and had to represent myself.

I tried to sue thirteen doctors. I had to pay $100 each to file the paperwork to sue each doctor, but of course, my poor ass did not have $1,300. My father said he could give me $300, so I sued Dr. Hoffman, Dr. Blackman, and Charity Hospital. I understood that the lawyers for the state based their strategy on the Statute of Limitations Legislative Act. The case should be dismissed because I had waited too long to sue the doctors. So, I had no legal right to sue.

But my strategy was simple, too; it was not my fault. It took me seven years to discover what was wrong with me. I knew I would tell the judge how I tried to shove information in front of those doctors, but they kept saying I had a physiological sickness.

On my court date, I went to court alone. The courtroom was packed with lawyers. I was so scared. The judge called my case. I went up to a long desk with my documents on plain notebook paper; the state lawyer was less than ten feet away from me at the desk, and everything went so fast.

The judge and the state lawyer said something, and they both looked at me. I said, "I have a rare disorder, and these doctors said I did not have it."

The judge stopped me and said, "That's not why we are here today." I just stood there.

The judge said something else, banged her gavel down, and told me I could leave the courtroom. I had to wait for the state lawyer to come out of the courtroom so I could find out what had just happened.

When she came out, I asked, "What happens now?"

"You go on with your life," she told me. "The judge ruled in the state's favor. It's not worth fighting. That's why you don't have a lawyer. Even if we went to court, you wouldn't get much; you must pay your lawyer. You can appeal, but it would be a waste of your time."

I cried because I had to face the fact that I was not getting my day in court.

I felt like something criminal had been done to me by the medical field. A jury of my peers needed to hear what happened and decide whether these doctors should compensate me for my pain and suffering. I wanted to tell the court about the psychiatrist misdiagnosing me with chemical imbalances I did not have, the one who wanted to take me to court to make me take psychiatric medication. I honestly wanted more than financial compensation; this was scary.

Even when they were wrong, doctors have power. Doctors have resources that regular people cannot access. It took me seven years to discover what a doctor could have discovered in seven months, seven days, or seven minutes. Doctors could ask their medical assistants to look up specific information. Doctors know what to look for when researching. I had to do it all myself.

After the court loss, I realized I was thirty years old, I had a condition that made me smell bad, and there was no cure. Even with a strict diet and exercise, the odor was always there. Deep down inside of me, I wished a magic pill could stop the odor forever. I was poor; I had two kids and did not know what to do. I was completely lost. I had a nervous breakdown that day in the courtroom, but I suppressed my feelings until April of 2004.

I was working as a housekeeper at a hotel. When I got off work, I went to the gym. I had only been a member of this particular gym for one month. I was working out, and a gym employee was speaking with another woman patron. The employee told the woman that some gym members complained that the steam room smelled like rotten fish. Of course, I used the steam room regularly, and I was an expert at knowing when people were talking about me, and I knew this bitch was talking about me. I immediately left the gym. I did not want to hear people talking about fish and smells. I got off the bus close to my neighborhood to walk and cry. I did not want to go home and cry in front of my son, who was at home with his father. I was glad that my daughter was at my aunt's house for a few days. My daughter could always look at my face and see when I had been crying. I had mistakenly told her after the TMAU diagnosis that I would be happy and not cry anymore.

I wiped my tears, and when I got into the house, my son ran up, hugged me, and said, "Mommy!" I hugged him back and sat down on the couch. As I sat there, my heart started racing. I jumped up and ran to get a cup of water. I thought, *I'm having a panic attack*, but it was different this time. My heart was racing, and I was sweating. I could not stop thinking about what the gym employee had said and about how I couldn't even sue the doctors. I had all these different thoughts going through my mind all at once. I felt like I couldn't breathe.

Corey Sr. asked, "What's wrong with you?"

"I do not know," I said as I ran from the kitchen to the bedroom. "Sit down. I will get you some water," he said.

I sat down, but I jumped right back up. I ran into the kitchen and Corey handed me the water. I gulped water and tried to breathe slowly but could not calm down.

My son was crying and asking, "Mama, why do you keep walking back and forth?"

I ran outside and down the stairs. I grabbed the banister to stop myself from running off the porch. I thought I would rip my clothes off and run down the street. Those thoughts were going through my mind as I stood on the porch. I knew what I was doing, but I could not stop walking. I was begging God, "Help me, Lord. Please do not let me lose my mind."

I returned to the house and told Corey to call an ambulance.

He said, "Just sit down." I ran into the kitchen.

I could see the knife on the counter. I thought of cutting my wrist with a knife. When I looked out the window, I thought of jumping out, but I stayed on the fourth floor. Corey Sr. came into the kitchen and grabbed my shoulders.

"Carry, you are scaring Corey Jr. Just sit down."

Corey Sr. had seen me have minor panic attacks before, but I kept trying to tell him this feeling was different. I asked him if he had called an ambulance.

"Yeah, they're on their way."

The ambulance pulled up. I walked to it.

The door opened, and the paramedic said, "Are you the person who called the ambulance?"

I said yes.

The paramedic asked me what was wrong as I got into the ambulance. I told them I thought I was having a panic attack but felt like I was losing my mind. I told the paramedics that my heart was racing, and I could not calm down.

They checked my vital signs. "Everything is normal. How do you feel right now?" they asked.

I told them I felt a little calmer.

"You just had a panic attack. Just go lie down. "It will pass," they said. Corey Sr. woke me up in the morning and said he had to leave.

I asked him, "Where is Corey Jr.?"

He replied, "Watching TV on the couch."

After Corey left, I got up.

My son said, "Mama, make me some cereal." I went into the kitchen and boiled some water to make coffee. I made cereal for Corey Jr. and got myself a cup of coffee. As I drank my coffee, I felt my heart racing. I started having uncontrollable thoughts again. I did not run to the bathroom. I did not want to scare my son. I took my clothes off and jumped in the shower, trying to cool myself off, but the shower was not working. I could not stop thinking.

When I got out of the shower, I got Corey Jr. dressed and headed to the hospital. As we walked to the bus stop, I was still having uncontrollable thoughts. I was scared to cross the street because of the traffic, but we safely reached the hospital.

I told the emergency room nurse I was having a panic attack. "I can't calm down; I can't stop thinking," I said.

The nurse took me to a room and they ran some tests.

A few hours later, the doctor entered my room and asked how I felt. I told him, "Okay, right now."

He said my vitals were normal, and my EKG showed no heart attack. He informed me that I'd had a panic attack and should follow up with my primary care doctor as soon as possible.

"I had a panic attack? What causes a panic attack?" I asked.

"Are you worried about something? he replied. "There are a lot of reasons a person could have anxiety or panic attacks. Your doctor can give you more information on these conditions."

I thanked him and Corey Jr. and I went home. I got home but was not feeling well, so I fixed something for my son to eat and laid down.

My son was playing with toys in the other room while I was lying in bed. I heard the toys hitting the floor as if I were lying on the floor, right next to them, and every time Corey Jr. hit the toys on the floor, I jumped like someone had snuck up on me and said, "Boo!"

"Please stop making noise!" I yelled. My heart started racing again. I jumped out of bed and called my cousin Tammy, who lived next door. I asked her to watch my son while I went to the emergency room. It was late, so I let my son go to my cousin's house, and I decided not to go to the hospital until the morning.

I called my downstairs neighbor and asked if I could stay the night with him because I feared being alone.

He said, "Sure."

I slept on his couch and woke up sweating profusely during the night. I was shaking, but I was not cold. My face felt like it was hanging down on the floor. I did not know what was wrong with me, but I knew it was serious.

The following morning, as I rode the bus to a charity hospital, the attacks worsened and came more frequently. When I got to the emergency room, I did not calm down this time. There were too many people in the waiting room, and I felt anxious. I had to grab hold of the arm of the chair to keep myself from walking back and forth.

After waiting thirty minutes, I walked up to a nurse and said, "Look, I feel like I am going to hurt myself; I need to see a doctor right now!"

She asked me if I was suicidal.

I said, "When I have attacks, I feel suicidal."

She asked me my name and if I had ever been to the hospital before. I started having an attack and yelled at her, "I need help now!"

She took me into a room and they took me upstairs. It scared me to be in the psychiatric ward of a charity hospital. I had tried to sue the hospital, and I was worried any psychiatrist I saw in the ward would know this, but I needed help.

"How can I help you?" The psychiatrist asked.

I asked the psychiatrist to please listen to what I was saying. "I am not suicidal, but I keep having these episodes where I cannot calm down. My heart is racing, and I feel like I cannot breathe. While I feel like that, thoughts of suicide and depression go through my mind."

"Is this the first time you have felt like this?"

"No, I have had minor panic attacks for the last four years, but they were never this severe. I do not want you to say I am having a panic attack when it's some psychotic break from reality."

"Ms. Wilson, you are not going crazy. You are having a panic attack. I am going to give you a sedative (Lorazepam) that will help to calm you down."

I shook my head. "No. I am not taking psychiatric drugs."

"Ms. Wilson, this pill is not an antipsychotic drug. This medicine will stop your heart and mind from racing. You will feel relaxed. If you were having surgery and you were nervous, this is the pill the doctor could give you to help you calm down and relax."

I did not want to keep running back and forth to the hospital, but it scared me to take the pills.

He said, "You can take one here just to see how you react."

When the nurse called me, I went up to her. She handed me the pill and a cup of water, and I started crying as I looked at the pill.

The nurse asked, "What's wrong?"

"I am scared to take this pill," I said.

"It's just going to make you feel calm," she told me.

"I am scared it will turn me into a zombie. Will I be aware of what is going on around me?" I asked.

"See how scared you are, and you said you cannot calm down, right?" she asked. "Take the lorazepam, and you will be calm."

I tried to put the pill in my mouth but could not.

A patient waiting to see a psychiatrist heard the nurse say the name of the pill and told me, "Girl, on the streets, they call them pills oral marijuana. I wish I were getting them."

After about twenty minutes, I finally took the pill. I sat down, and within minutes, a calm, warm feeling came over my body. I felt relaxed. I was at ease. The doctor called me to the counter, and as I walked toward him, I felt like I was walking on air. The doctor asked me how I felt.

In a whisper, I said," I feel okay."

"I will give you a prescription for some more pills, but I want you to make an appointment with a psychiatrist," he said.

When I left the hospital and stepped outside, the wind felt good against my skin. I thought the day I tested positive for TMAU was when I changed emotionally, but that day, in that moment, I felt better than I had in seven years. The guy on the bus talked to me about how long buses took to arrive. I was always quiet on the bus, but the pill made me not care what other people thought of me.

I still have anxiety and panic attacks. The sedative I took was a momentary fix for my symptoms. Anyone having anxiety or panic attacks should seek treatment with a healthcare professional.

THE END

Finally, in 2023, I stopped trying to find a cure for Trimethylaminuria/Fish Odor Syndrome (TMAU) in the supplement aisle of my local pharmacy. There is no cure right now. I am focused on treatment and my mental health. I said I would never take any psychiatric medication. I now take psychiatric medication (antidepressants) and probably will have to for the rest of my life. Those seven years I went undiagnosed have defined my psychological health. I have truly accepted that I have a medical condition that causes my body to have a foul odor. I will do everything I can to get and keep my body odor level down to undetectable levels. It isn't easy, but I will never give up.

Not every person who has body odor has TMAU. They may have another condition. A person should never want to kill themselves because they smell bad. When we go to work, our coworkers make vicious comments about those of us with body odor. When we go shopping, people make disrespectful comments about our body odor. We must remember that we have a rare medical condition. It is not normal to smell foul, and some people do not just smell the way they smell; there is always a reason. If you cannot keep a job because you feel humiliated or suffer from depression, apply for financial disability if you consider this an option. Sufferers of body odor have the right to a workplace that is not a hostile environment.

I can honestly say that I understand why people don't want

to go to work and smell the scent of feces or rotten fish; however, those of us with body odor don't want to smell like rotten fish, and we must earn a living just like everyone else. I did not want to be on disability initially, but I needed it to survive. Talk to your supervisor at work if you are being harassed by your coworkers about your body odor and see if they can give you a work assignment that lessens your contact with your coworkers. People with body odor can work wherever and with whomever they want. People with body odor may need to change their lifestyles to live a half-normal life. Eat healthy and exercise. People assume that people with body odors are not clean. However, we are the cleanest people on the planet because we must be.

Dr. Pratt once told me that TMAU is a high-maintenance condition to care for. Not only was he right, but it's also an understatement. We have a plan we want to fulfill. Body odor does not stop us from achieving or wanting goals. We want to own a home, have a business, and have a 401k plan. (What exactly is a 401k plan?) I will pray for the rest of my life for a cure for body odor conditions. I will pray to be successful enough to own a home where I can build a steam or sauna room, which do wonders for body odor levels and my mental state of mind.

Please dress cleanly, groom your hair, and care about your appearance. I smelled horrible, and I looked awful. Remember, we have this condition; the condition does not have us. If you are being harassed at work because of your disability or body odor, call for information on the Americans with Disabilities Act or your local rehabilitation services for people with disabilities.

Organic things I do to keep my body odor levels down:
I will try not to go too far with advice. We are all different, and what works for one person may not work for another. It would help if you always collaborated with your doctor when adding and eliminating foods from your diet or starting a workout routine.

Exercising

Exercising is the most organic activity you can do to help reduce your body odor and increase your health simultaneously. I exercise three to five days a week, concentrating on cardio. I aim to build up enough sweat at least three times a week during my workouts to sweat heavily, which reduces my body odor. After working out, I sit in a steam room or dry sauna for fifteen minutes. At the end of my workout, I feel like I have naturally detoxed all the toxins out of my body.

Diet/Lifestyle Change

Dieting must become a lifestyle change for body odor sufferers. I have found that a lot of the food that is healthy for most people is a trigger for TMAU. I must choose: do I eat green vegetables sometimes or cut them out of my diet completely? I decided it was beneficial to my health to include green vegetables like broccoli, kale, and spinach, as well as other vegetables and plant-based foods, at least twice a month in my diet. But these foods will increase my body odor. I enjoy eating foods that are heart, bone, and brain healthy. I eat a lot of bland food. No heavy salt, seasonings, or condiments like ketchup, mustard, etc. I eat whole-grain wheat products, probiotic yogurts, and fermented foods in moderation. Fermented foods are natural probiotics.

Treatment

I treat my body odor with diet, exercise, and probiotics. In 2020, I was on YouTube. I found a great channel, the Gut War! This guy has a lot of brilliant advice on food, kefir, and kombucha as treatment options for TMAU. Probiotics are an important ingredient in kombucha and kefir. These products have shown impressive results for some people with TMAU.

I talked to my doctor and was told I could try kombucha and kefir. This was the first time in over 20 years I have taken advice about TMAU treatment options. I drank two cups of pre-made kombucha daily and got satisfactory results. I take probiotic and prebiotic supplements once a day. I will drink a bottle of kefir or kombucha as desired.

Do your homework. There are many probiotics with different strains, some with good anecdotal results. I like the Walgreen Drug Store's probiotic brand. I have had significant results with their strain of probiotics.

Talk with your doctor, and you might consider probiotics as an option to treat your TMAU. Educate yourself on how better gut health can be directly beneficial to treating TMAU and other body odor conditions. Better gut health could be life changing.

Survival, family, happiness, love, and life

Talk to your doctor and seek professional help if you have depression or are experiencing symptoms of depression. Eat healthier, exercise, and investigate the pros and cons of taking probiotics. Remember, you always know the odor is there, but sometimes other people may not smell you when you think they can. Everyone is different. You must get to know your body and learn how to control your body odor. Some people with body odor may find it challenging to get their body odor levels down, but you must keep trying. It is a slow process, but it is worth it. We deserve life, love, and happiness, too.

My YouTube Channel: Carry Wilson-TMAU.

If you or someone you know has a body odor and would like to get tested, received information on conditions with body odor as a symptom, or learn about your rights to work with a body odor condition.

Call or write:
NORD (The National Organization of Rare Disorders)
617-249-7300

The Children's Hospital of Colorado

720-777-6711

Americans with Disability Act (Civil Rights Division)
800-514-0301
Please email me with questions: godcarrywilson@yahoo.com

APPENDIX

July 1997

Chicago Illinois

This is the first medical record of my journey through the Psychological, psychiatric experience.

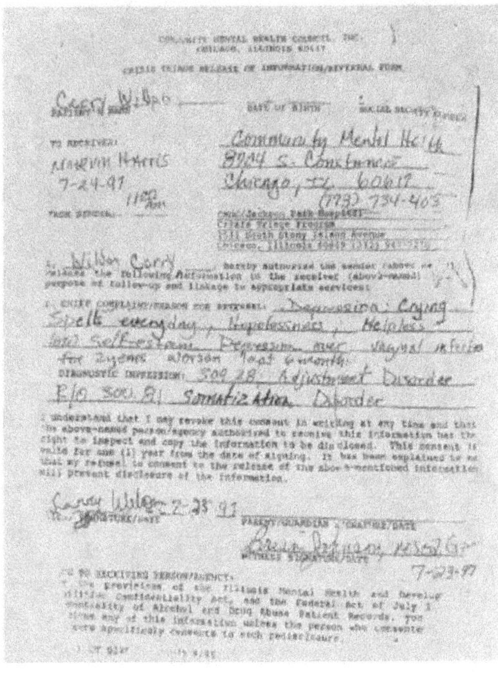
COMMUNITY MENTAL HEALTH COUNCIL, INC.
CHICAGO, ILLINOIS [illegible]

CRISIS TRIAGE RELEASE OF INFORMATION/REFERRAL FORM

Carry Wilson
PATIENT'S NAME — DATE OF BIRTH — SOCIAL SECURITY NUMBER

TO RECEIVER: Community Mental Health
8704 S. Constance
Chicago, IL 60617
(773) 734-405[illegible]

Marvin Harris
7-24-97
11:00 AM

FROM SENDER: [illegible]/Jackson Park Hospital
Crisis Triage Program
[illegible] South Stony Island Avenue
Chicago, Illinois [illegible]

I, Wilson Carry, hereby authorize the sender (above) to release the following information to the receiver (above-named) for purpose of follow-up and linkage to appropriate services:

CHIEF COMPLAINT/REASON FOR REFERRAL: Depression; Crying spells everyday, hopelessness, helpless, low self-esteem. Depression over vaginal infection for 2 years, abortion last 6 months.

DIAGNOSTIC IMPRESSION: 309.28 Adjustment Disorder
R/O 300.81 Somatization Disorder

I understand that I may revoke this consent in writing at any time and that the above-named person/agency authorized to receive this information has the right to inspect and copy the information to be disclosed. This consent is valid for one (1) year from the date of signing. It has been explained to me that my refusal to consent to the release of the above-mentioned information will prevent disclosure of the information.

Carry Wilson 7-23-97
SIGNATURE/DATE

PARENT/GUARDIAN SIGNATURE/DATE

[illegible] Johnson, [illegible]
WITNESS SIGNATURE/DATE
7-23-97

Part 1

1998-2001

New Orleans Louisiana

I resorted to altering my medical records. I did not want any new doctors I saw to read the statement "No odor appreciated". Not only that, I used whiteout and copy and paste to alter my records. (Still no help)

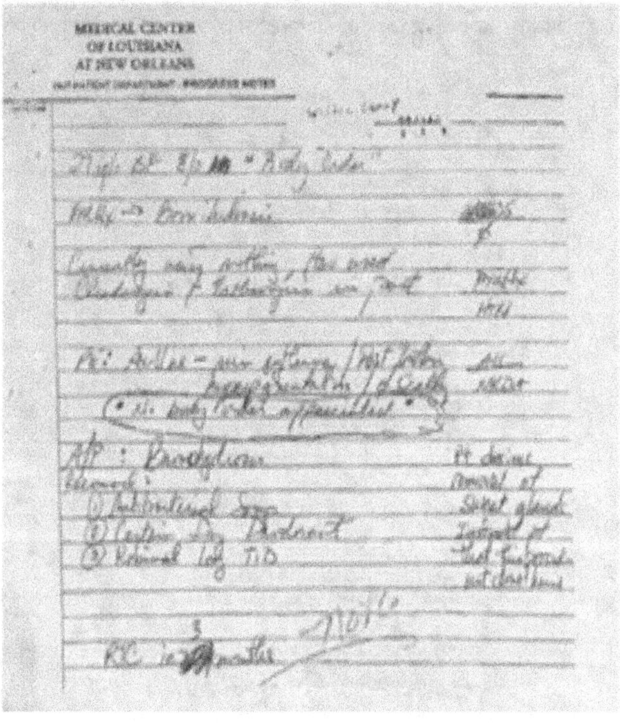

MEDICAL CENTER
OF LOUISIANA
AT NEW ORLEANS

Part 2

New Orleans Louisa

1998-2001

This is one of my altered medical records that I used white-out on.

I removed the statement (No body odor appreciated)

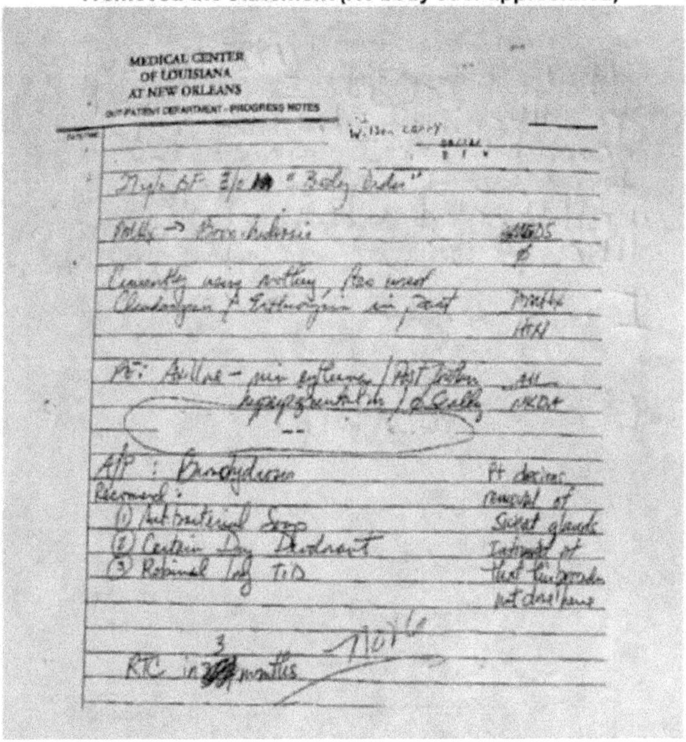

MEDICAL CENTER
OF LOUISIANA
AT NEW ORLEANS
OUT-PATIENT DEPARTMENT - PROGRESS NOTES

Recommend:
(1) Antibacterial Soap
(2) Certain Dry Deodorant
(3) Robinul 1mg TID

RTC in 3 months

Part 1

October 2001

New Orleans Louisiana

I altered my medical record. I did not want any new doctors I saw to see the word Phobia charted on my record.

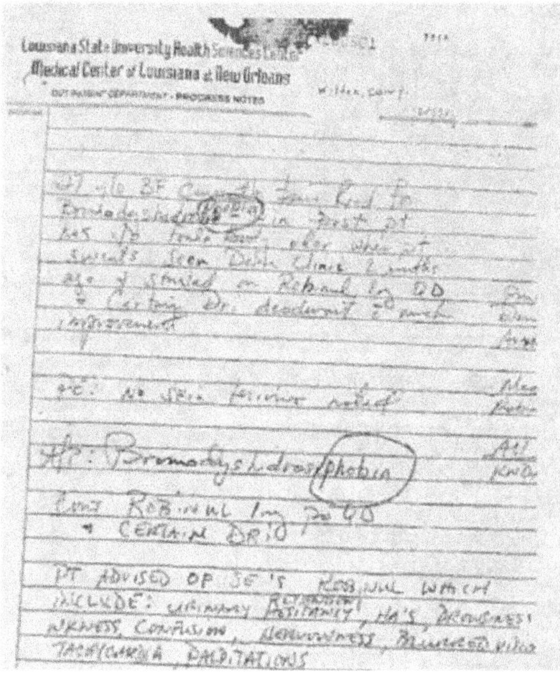

Part 2

October 2001
New Orleans Louisiana

I used whiteout and changed the word Bromhidrosisphobia to Bromhidrosis

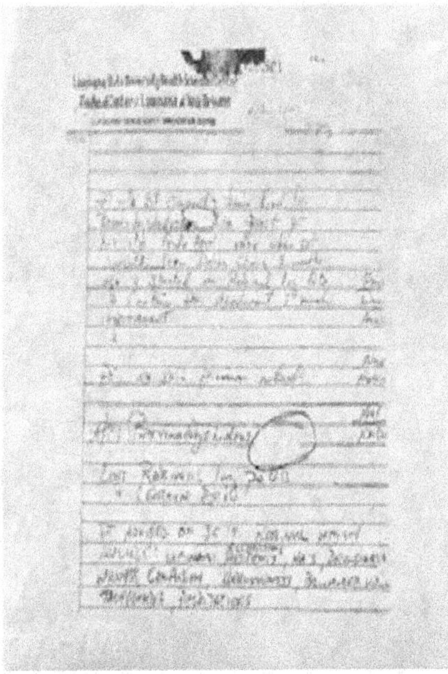

2003

New Orleans, Louisiana

Medical invoice record of surgeons in Chicago, IL, who were going to perform the sweat gland surgery removal for two thousand nine hundred and ninety-seven dollars (2997.00)

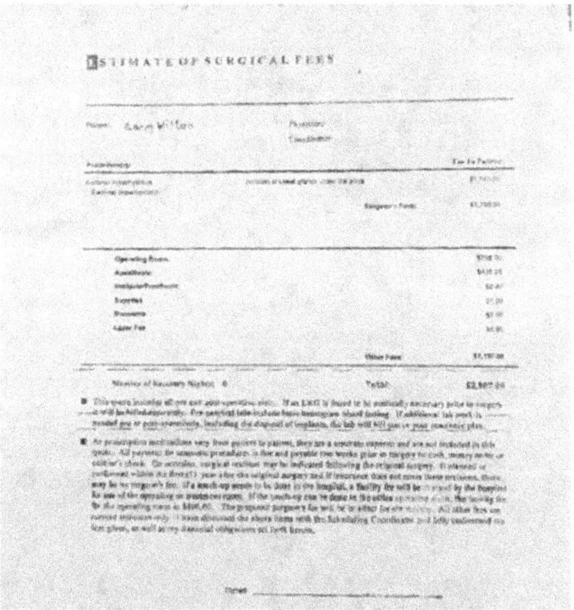

ESTIMATE OF SURGICAL FEES

Operating Room

Supplies

Laser Fee

Total:

March 2003

New Orleans Louisiana

Statement at the bottom of this document, lead to me getting tested for Trimethylaminuria (TMAU) old name was Fish Odor Syndrome

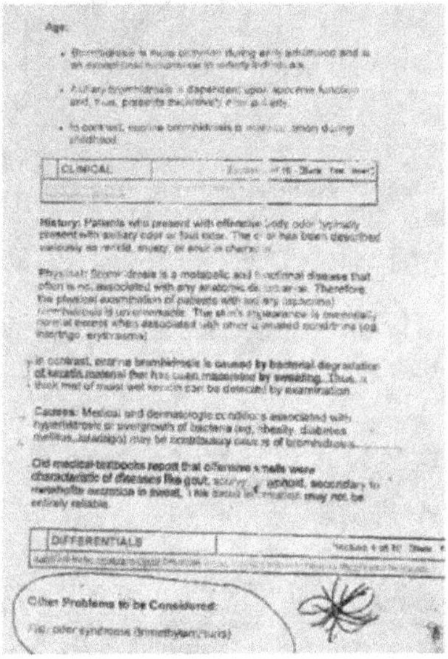

Age:

- Bromhidrosis is more common during early adulthood and is an exceptional occurrence in elderly individuals.
- Axillary bromhidrosis is dependent upon apocrine function and, thus, presents exclusively after puberty.
- In contrast, eccrine bromhidrosis is [illegible] during childhood.

	CLINICAL	[illegible]

History: Patients who present with offensive body odor typically present with axillary odor or foul feet. The odor has been described variously as rancid, musty, or [illegible] in character.

Physical: Bromhidrosis is a metabolic and functional disease that often is not associated with any anatomic [illegible]. Therefore, the physical examination of patients with axillary (apocrine) bromhidrosis is unremarkable. The skin's appearance is essentially normal except when associated with other [illegible] conditions (eg, intertrigo, erythrasma).

In contrast, eccrine bromhidrosis is caused by bacterial degradation of keratin material that has been macerated by sweating. Thus, a thick mat of moist wet keratin can be detected by examination.

Causes: Medical and dermatologic conditions associated with hyperhidrosis or overgrowth of bacteria (eg, obesity, diabetes mellitus, intertrigo) may be contributory causes of bromhidrosis.

Old medical textbooks report that offensive smells were characteristic of diseases like gout, scurvy, [illegible], secondary to metabolite excretion in sweat. This [illegible] information may not be entirely reliable.

	DIFFERENTIALS	[illegible]

Other Problems to be Considered:

Fish odor syndrome (trimethylaminuria)

March 2003

1 of only 6 informational documents that NORD sent me in 2003 on Trimethylaminuria

In 2003, there was limited information on trimethylaminuria

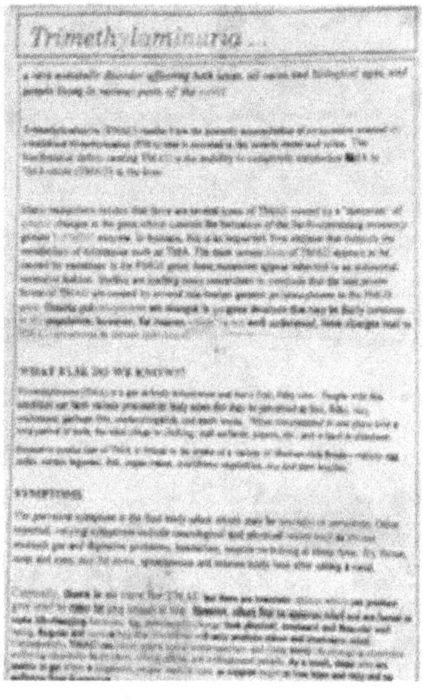

2003

2 of 6 informational documents on TMAU

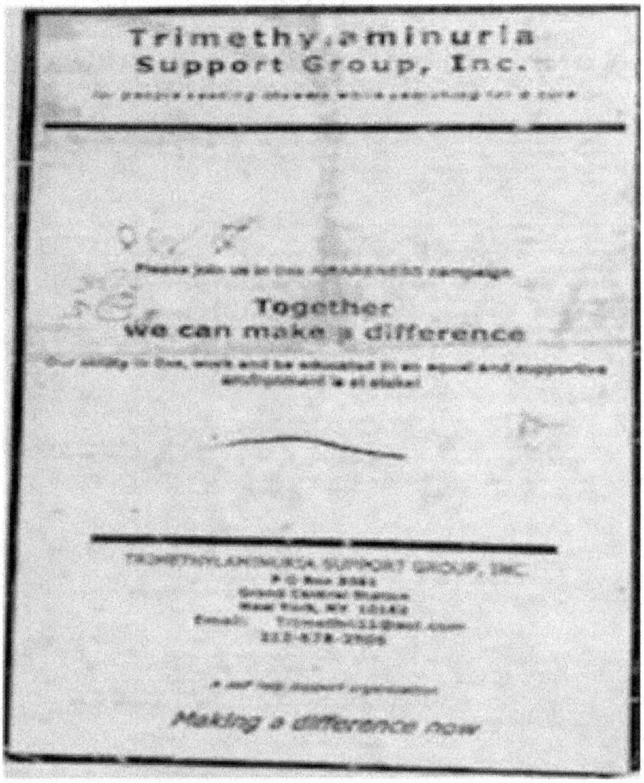
Trimethylaminuria
Support Group, Inc.

Together
we can make a difference

Making a difference now

2003

3 of 6 informational documents on TMAU

2003

4 of 6 informational documents on TMAU

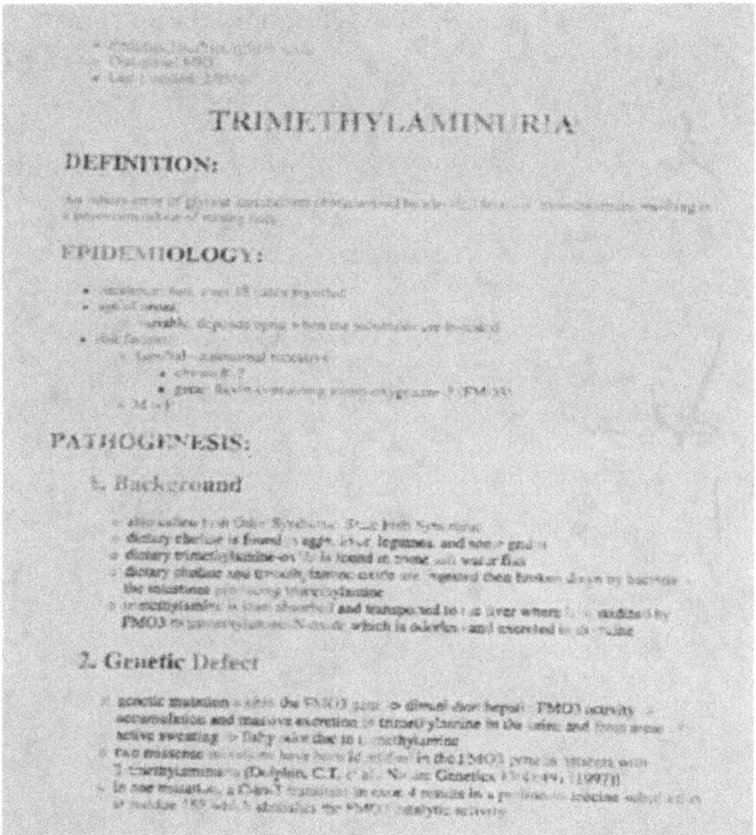

TRIMETHYLAMINURIA

DEFINITION:

EPIDEMIOLOGY:

PATHOGENESIS:

1. Background

2. Genetic Defect

2003

5 of 6 informational documents on TMAU

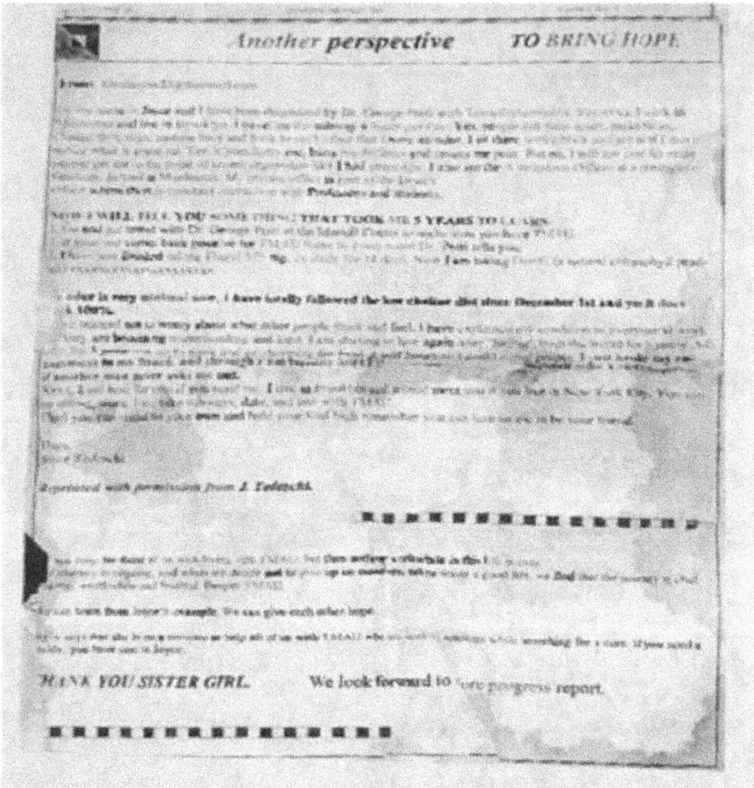

Another perspective *TO BRING HOPE*

Reprinted with permission from J. Tedeschi.

THANK YOU SISTER GIRL. We look forward to more progress report.

2003

6 of 6 informational documents on TMAU

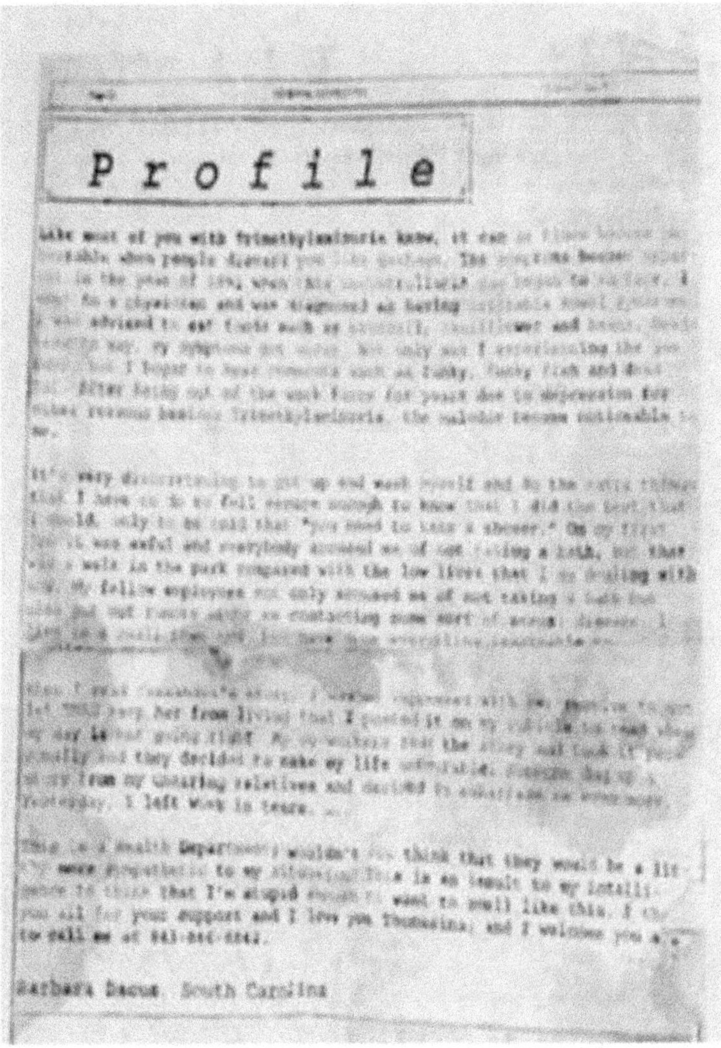

Profile

April 2003

Part 1: The letter

New Orleans

Letter I wrote to the late Dr. George Preti to start the TMAU testing process. I felt the need to state in the letter that doctors had given me good hygiene advice. I did not want Dr. Preti to know that my interactions with doctors have been less than helpful. I did not receive good hygiene advice from doctors.

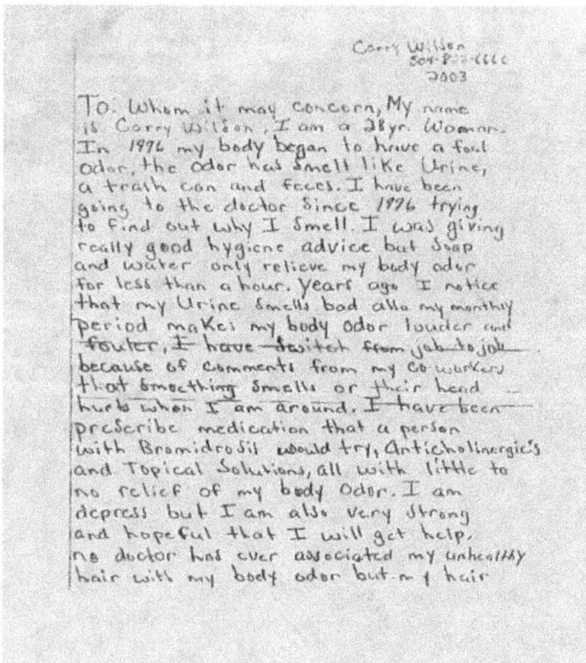

Carry Wilson
504-[illegible]
2003

To: Whom it may concern, My name is Carry Wilson, I am a 28yr. Woman. In 1996 my body began to have a foul odor, the odor has smell like Urine, a trash can and feces. I have been going to the doctor since 1996 trying to find out why I smell. I was giving really good hygiene advice but soap and water only relieve my body odor for less than a hour. Years ago I notice that my Urine smells bad also my monthly period makes my body odor louder and fouler, I have switch from job to job because of comments from my co-workers that something smells or their head hurts when I am around. I have been prescribe medication that a person with Bromidrosis would try, Anticholinergic's and Topical Solutions, all with little to no relief of my body odor. I am depress but I am also very strong and hopeful that I will get help. no doctor has ever associated my unhealthy hair with my body odor but my hair

May 2003

New Orleans Louisiana

My POSITIVE test results for TMAU

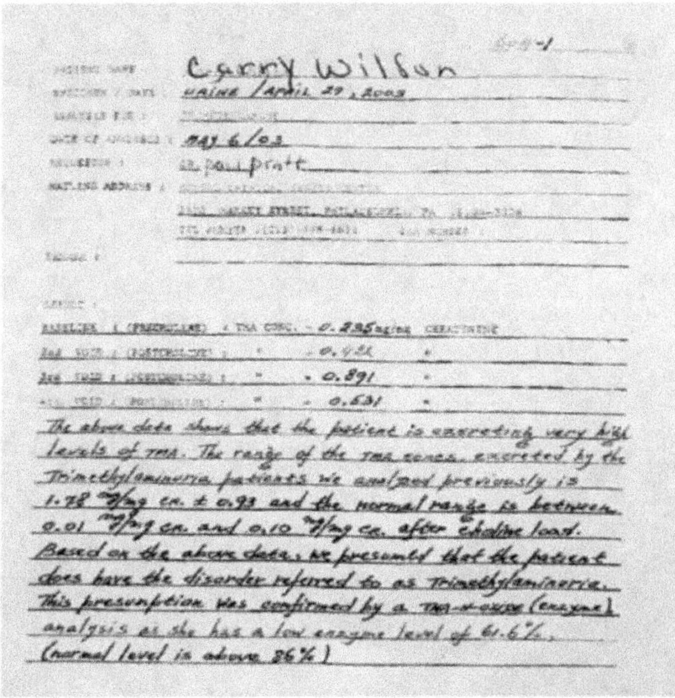

Garry Willson

urine / April 29, 2003

May 6/03

dr. paul pratt

0.295 mg/mg creatinine

0.491

0.891

0.531

The above data shows that the patient is excreting very high levels of TMA. The range of the TMA conc. excreted by the Trimethylaminuria patients we analyzed previously is 1.78 mg/mg cr. ± 0.93 and the normal range is between 0.01 mg/mg cr. and 0.10 mg/mg cr. after choline load. Based on the above data, we presume that the patient does have the disorder referred to as Trimethylaminuria. This presumption was confirmed by a TMA-N-oxide (enzyme) analysis as she has a low enzyme level of 61.6%. (normal level is above 86%)